THE
Saint
Tropez
Diet

Look your best. Feel your best. Love what you eat.

THE
Saint
Tropez
Diet

Apostolos Pappas, Ph.D.
with Marie-Annick Courtier

HATHERLEIGH PRESS

New York • London

HATHERLEIGH PRESS

5-22 46th Avenue, Suite 200
Long Island City, NY 11101
www.hatherleighpress.com
www.SaintTropezDiet.com

DISCLAIMER

The ideas and suggestions contained in this book are not intended as a
substitute for consulting with a physician. All matters regarding your health
require medical supervision.

Library of Congress Cataloging-in-Publication Data
Pappas, Apostolos.
  The Saint-Tropez diet : unlock the secrets of the French Riviera for a slimmer, sexier, and
healthier you / Apostolos Pappas and Marie-Annick Courtier.
     p. cm.
  Includes index.
  ISBN 1-57826-235-6
  1. Nutrition--France--Saint-Tropez. 2. Diet—France—Saint-Tropez. 3.
Cookery—France—Saint-Tropez. I. Courtier, Marie-Annick. II. Title.
  RA784.P336 2007
  613.2'5—dc22
                            2006036567
  ISBN-13: 978-1-57826-235-9
  ISBN-10: 1-57826-235-6

Interior design by Christine Weathersbee, Deborah Miller, Allison Furrer, Jasmine Cordoza
Interior photos by Brand X Pictures®, Getty Images® and Apostolos Pappas
Cover illustration by Getty Images®
Cover design by Deborah Miller
Cover photos by Apostolos Pappas

10 9 8 7 6 5 4 3 2 1
Printed in the United States

Acknowledgments

We would like to thank everyone at Hatherleigh Press who worked so hard and made this book possible, including publisher Kevin Moran, editorial director Andrea Au, and art director Deborah Miller, and especially the mastermind behind this book, Andrew Flach. In addition, many thanks to writer Michelle Seaton for her magic touch on the text and to Tracy Olgeaty Gensler, M.S., R.D., for her help with the meal plans.

Dedication

To my graduate school mentors, Drs. S. M. Constantinides and G. M. Carman, my parents and family in Greece, and my French godchild Camille in Lausanne.

—Apostolos

To my family, friends, and Chef Al, who all contributed to my true passion for healthy cuisine.

—Marie

Contents

Introduction

Although I have always had a passion for both food and wine, I have a particular obsession with chocolate. In fact, my American colleagues have often wondered aloud to me how it can be possible for me to eat chocolate every day without getting fat. What is my secret, they ask. To a food scientist, this is not the simple question that it seems to be. Perhaps my research has been leading me to try and answer this very question. Is there a diet that will allow for moderate sweets and even wine that will still promote weight loss and good health? I would find many of these answers in my research.

From the very beginning of my career I have had to swing between my course curriculum in food science, which is the scientific study of everything related to food, and my core research projects in biochemistry, which is the study of—among other things—what happens to food once it enters the body. In particular, biochemistry studies how the cells make use of nutrients. Much of my research has focused on how the skin cells make use of fats. Through my research I found myself studying the ways in which the body metabolizes fat and in particular how it makes use of fatty acids.

The study of fatty acids has exploded in recent years, much to the benefit of both food scientists and dietitians. Modern instrumentation and better analytical techniques have shown how these fatty acids interact with our DNA. This same body of research has revealed new molecules called nutraceuticals, which also interact with our genetic material. Apparently, all these nutrients are ample in the foods I grew up eating in Greece, a diet that most people still believe is the healthiest in the world. I began to wonder if this new research could actually improve upon the Mediterranean diet so that it would promote greater health and stimulate weight loss.

My own observations of different diets seemed to support this. My study and research kept me in the United States for a long time, where I had to become used to convenience foods, highly processed grains, and even snack foods such as chips and sodas. Then in 2001, I returned to Europe where I stayed for two years. I spent time in different parts of both Germany and France, where I closely observed the diet of my colleagues and the people around me. It became more apparent to me that people in Europe eat differently. They cook more and snack less. While they do not necessarily eat less, and they spend far less time in a gym, they are more active in their day-to-day activities. What is striking is that most people in Europe can easily maintain a healthy weight without counting calories or grams of fat.

Upon my return to the United States in 2003, I kept observing the diets and lifestyles around me. My friends and colleagues were always conscious about their diet, always counting calories, and cutting either fat or carbohydrates. Still, they gained weight or failed to lose weight. It struck me that they overlooked profound attributes, such as the quality of fat and the wholesomeness of their food. They claimed to love good-tasting food but continually reached for flat-tasting breads and pastas and fast foods that to me tasted like nothing. I thought this could be a piece of the puzzle.

In recent years, I've traveled several times to Saint-Tropez, a place where I could find food similar to that which I enjoyed in my early years in Greece. I ate fresh fish, olive oil, and nuts that contained the healthiest fats together with the richest variety of vegetables and fruit. I even drank wine and ate chocolate. All around me, people enjoyed gourmet food and great health. A lifelong Francophile, I knew I'd found the right place. Those trips, together with my observations and research over the years, inspired the Saint-Tropez Diet. With this book, including the delicious recipes by Chef Marie and other renowned French chefs, I hope to inspire you all to eat as the people of Saint-Tropez do, following the healthiest diet in the world.

—*Apostolos Pappas, Ph.D.*
August 2006

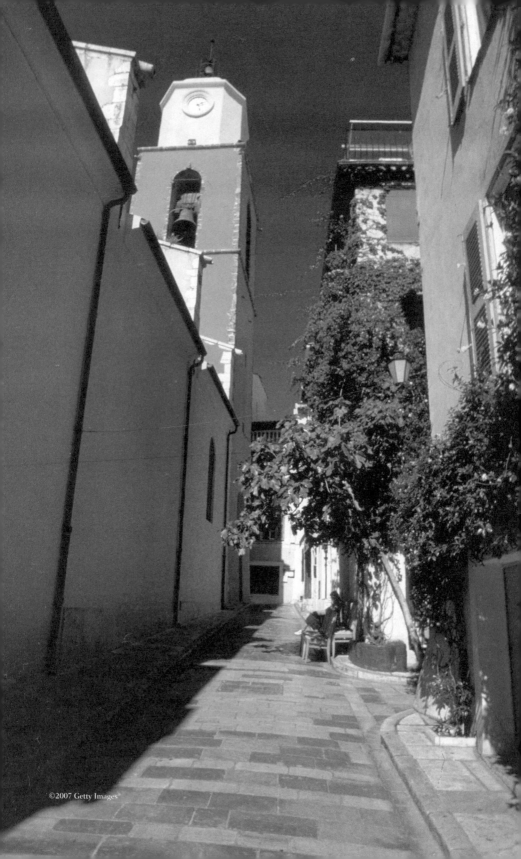

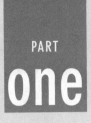

PART

one

Principles of the Saint-Tropez Diet

The Saint-Tropez Diet is more than just a weight loss plan. It is a way of eating that emulates the Mediterranean and French diets—the two healthiest diets in the world—in order to make you slimmer, healthier, and more energetic.

By increasing the amount of fresh foods and healthy fats in your diet—as well as slightly reducing the number of calories you eat—you can reap all of the weight loss benefits of this diet while feeling full and satisfied after each meal. By learning how to combine foods to maximum effect, you can supercharge your metabolism and further increase the health benefits of this diet to improve your skin tone, your blood sugar levels, your arteries, and even your mood.

In these first few chapters, you'll learn why the people of Saint-Tropez have the best possible diet. You'll learn why eating the right kind of fat can actually increase your body's tendency to burn fat. You'll discover which foods contain hidden health benefits, and which myths about dieting can ruin your efforts to lose weight. You'll even learn why a small amount of wine will never interfere with your good health or your efforts to maintain a slender waistline.

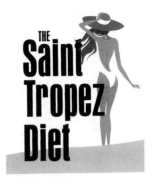

Welcome to Saint-Tropez

The cities and beach communities along the southern shore of Provence have long been known collectively as the Côte d'Azur, or the Azure Coast, for the endlessly blue skies over the ocean. Several of these cities, such as Nice and Cannes, have been famous vacation spots for the rich and famous since the late 1800s.

Until the 1950s, Saint-Tropez was the exception, a sleepy fishing village ignored by tourists. Now it has become one of the most glamorous vacation spots in the world, a fact that still puzzles the 5,000 or so local residents. The town itself is so close to the ocean that it seems perched on top of it. In fact, for centuries the port town was only readily accessible by boat because of its location out on the bay of Saint-Tropez. Given the constant traffic jams on the narrow roads leading to town, this may still be true.

In the 1880s, novelist Guy de Maupassant sailed his yacht into the harbor of Saint-Tropez and found it a haven for his ailing body and spirit. In his short story "Sur L'Eau," he described Saint-Tropez as "looking like a seashell, wet from the saltwater and nourished by the fish and sea air."

The hills and cliffs surrounding the town offer beautiful views of the ocean and beaches, which are particularly stunning during sunrises and sunsets. These views, as well as the quiet nature of the village itself, attracted many impressionistic painters at the turn of the twentieth century, including Paul Signac and Henry Matisse. In the 1930s, the writers arrived, including Anaïs Nin. It's no surprise that she was drawn to the sexual freedom she saw all around. Nin described the nude women riding in cars with their rich boyfriends. In

Prisons et Paradis, Colette wrote of a different kind of freedom. She found an embracing warmth in Saint-Tropez that encouraged her to discover herself. Then Jean-Paul Sartre, Simon de Beauvoir, and Jacques Prevert turned it into a summertime Left Bank. Suddenly liberated from Paris's stifling summer heat, these writers would spend

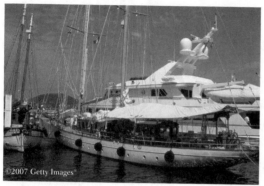

whole afternoons at the cafes facing the bay watching the eerie blue waters or the locals walking by. Even now, sitting in one of those cafes and watching the mega-yachts or the tourists strolling by is a day-long activity for some.

Saint-Tropez remained a sleepy village, a haven for bo-hemian artists through two World Wars. Then in 1956, Brigitte Bardot arrived to film *And God Created Woman*, in which she sunbathed nude and had affairs with three different men. The film made both Bardot and Saint-Tropez instantly famous for their striking beauty and casual sensuality. The next year, the American production *The Vintage*, starring Mel Ferrer and Michelle Morgan, portrayed an earthy, forbidden love affair filled with wine and the great flavors of the region. In the 1960s, the master of French film noir, Claude Chabrol, chose Saint-Tropez as a setting for several of his movies. In *Les Biches*, he depicted a perplexed love triangle made glamorous by the breathtaking backdrop of the Saint-Tropez lifestyle. In the same year, 1968, the four participants in the "love square" in *La Piscine* spent their vacation in a villa near Saint-Tropez and made millions of moviegoers dream about doing the same.

The Saint-Tropez mystique was fueled further by the *Le Gendarme de St. Tropez* series of films, in which the great French comedian Louis de Funès played ambitious police officer Cruchot whose teenage daughter tries to impress her rich friends by telling them her father is a millionaire who owns a yacht—but of course the real yacht owners aren't exactly what they pretend to be either.... Similarly, the high camp of *La Cage Aux Folles* in the late 1970s could not have been filmed anywhere else but in "Saint-Tropez, the capital of the rich and famous," as it was loudly proclaimed in legendary French director Claude Lelouch's caustic social satire, *Smic Smac Smoc*.

Ever since, the town has drawn the richest and most famous people in the world, many of whom moor their yachts in the harbor and come ashore to shop by day and party at night. Some celebrities arrive by helicopter to carouse in the bars or join their friends at parties in the enormous villas on the outskirts of town. Uma Thurman, Paris Hilton, Bono, Bruce Willis, Sean "Diddy" Combs, Naomi Campbell, Donatella Versace, Ivana Trump, and David and Victoria Beckham are among the boldfaced names who have vacationed in Saint-Tropez in recent years.

This glamor belies the real charm and heart of this ancient port town. Those who visit Saint-Tropez in the off season, from September to May, can still find a rather small village of less than a square mile, with narrow streets, ancient architecture, and outdoor cafés featuring a cuisine that bears the influences of both Provence and the Mediterranean. Travelers who come build their days around the fabulous restaurants and spend time in between meals at the beach or

WHERE TO EAT IN SAINT-TROPEZ

If you are lucky enough to travel to Saint-Tropez, be sure to visit some of the trendiest restaurants where Hollywood celebrities, musicians, and artists like to eat. Among these is the gourmet Italian restaurant Villa Romana, located on the Chemin des Coquettes. The restaurant is famous for its homemade pasta with fish sauces, fresh seafood dishes, and truffles imported from Italy. The rich and famous in Saint-Tropez also like to dine at Joseph, a more formal restaurant that serves elaborate Mediterranean dishes. Its companion restaurant, Petit Joseph, serves Thai and Cambodian food. Several of the private beaches in Saint-Tropez rent lounge chairs and have small bistros at which they serve food. Among the best are Club 55, which is quite popular among billionaire residents even though it is open only for lunch—meaning from noon to 6 every day. The younger jet-setters in Saint-Tropez favor the club at Nikki Beach.

shopping at offbeat boutiques that line the narrow streets. Like the natives, they plan whole weeks around market days.

Market Days

Locals gather on the Place des Lices, a popular common in the heart of Saint-Tropez, to play boules, the French version of bocce—except on Tuesday and Saturday. On these days, vendors take over the area. Here, in a park shaded by plane trees, vendors set up canopies and umbrellas from which they sell fresh fruits and vegetables, breads, herbs, olives, and even homemade tapenades. The smell of fresh lavender and flowers permeates the entire market. The locals know to go early in the morning, before the tourists arrive, to buy produce for the week and to plan their meals according to which vegetables are in season and which are freshest. Buyers wend their way among

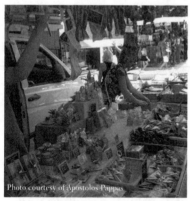

Photo courtesy of Apostolos Pappas

the stalls, reading the hand-lettered signs that mark the day's prices and chatting with the vendors they know well. It's a lively experience in which shopping is a social and sensual event.

When locals need to buy fish—which is nearly every day—they go to the Place aux Herbs, a square near the water, where there is a daily market for sellers of fruits, vegetables, and flowers. Here you can buy fish that was caught just hours ago, which is one of the reasons the seafood dishes in Saint-Tropez are so delicious and so pervasive. It is also one of the reasons why the locals are so healthy and so thin.

A Healthy, Fat-Burning Diet

In Saint-Tropez, locals live a life full of sensual pleasures. They enjoy the white beaches and sea air, the soft light and sublime weather. But they also have a special relationship with food, one that helps them to stay healthy and fit. Sure, they walk more than Americans do. They walk to market and to restaurants, and they walk after eating. But the key to their good health is their diet. In Provence, people love to cook and to shop for fresh ingredients, and they don't starve themselves to stay thin. They eat, and they love to eat.

The diet that has evolved here is one of the healthiest in the world, based primarily on fish and olive oil, augmented with fruits and vegetables, legumes and whole grains. Here in Saint-Tropez, the hearty Provençal fare—based as it is on garlic, olive oil, onions, herbs, tomatoes, potatoes, beans, lots of greens, fish, and some meats—takes these traditional Mediterranean ingredients and blends them with the French passion for layering textures and tastes creatively. If you spent enough time here, walking where the locals do, eating what they eat, and living as they live, you would lose weight, boost your energy levels, and slow down your aging process.

Even if you don't have a local farmer's market in which to shop every day, even if you don't have a fishmonger within walking distance of your home, you can still learn to cook and eat and love food in the exact same way that the people do here. When you do, you will find your waistline shrinking and your energy soaring.

In the next few chapters, you'll learn how to recreate the Saint-Tropez way of life in your own kitchen and change your diet for the better forever.

CHAPTER

2

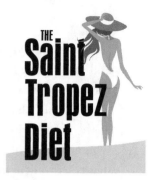

THE
Saint
Tropez
Diet

Improving on the Healthiest
Diet in the World

If you did travel to Saint-Tropez to enjoy the beaches and the great food, the first thing you would discover is that the food you were eating would be vastly different from the food you may be used to now. After all, Saint-Tropez is where the cuisine of France, especially Provence, meets the Mediterranean. These two types of cuisine are not only the most delicious, they also have important health benefits.

In 1986, Ansel Keys of the University of Minnesota and his colleagues from Italy, the Netherlands, Japan, Yugoslavia, Finland, and Greece published a study that had tracked the death rates of 12,000 study subjects in all of those countries (plus the United States), and found that the men in Greece, who took in the highest levels of olive oil and other monounsaturated fats, had the lowest rates of death from heart disease. For example, the study found that American men were 20 times more likely to die of heart disease and twice as likely to die of cancer as men on the Isle of Crete. These Greek men were far healthier and lived longer, despite the fact that they consumed a diet much higher in fat than the traditional American diet. In fact, their diet was comprised primarily of 40 percent fat in the form of olive oil cooked with vegetables and legumes. Even when the study corrected the raw data for certain lifestyle factors such as smoking, stress, and baseline body fat, there was a significant disparity between the men in Greece and those in every other culture in the study.

In the intervening decades, many studies have taken apart this diet in order to discover its secrets. First, scientists studied the olive oil.

Could that be a miracle food? Then a group of studies found that the French, who consume far more saturated fats than Americans, smoke more, and spend less time in rigorous exercise at gyms (although they walk more), still have a lower rate of death from heart disease. According to one study, the rate of death by heart disease in France is just one-third of that in the United States. This disparity became known as the French Paradox. Theories abounded to explain the paradox, including the notion that the tannins in red wine might have a positive health benefit. Subsequent studies on this have had mixed results. Alarmingly, newer studies are showing that the increase in junk food and fast food consumption in France may take away the natural health advantage they have so far enjoyed. In fact, several studies show that obesity is on the rise in many European countries, including France.

Finally, a group of studies conducted by Artemis Simopoulos, author of *The Omega Diet,* isolated one important fact: that the ratio of essential fatty acids in these diets is the key to their success. It is not just what people in France and Greece eat, but what they don't eat that matters. Dr. Simopoulos further postulated that mass production of certain food items in the West might be contributing to a decline in health. The American diet is loaded in white flour and corn oil, high in omega-6 essential fatty acids, while deficient in foods such as nuts and oily fish, which are high in omega-3 essential fatty acids. In addition, the Western diet is very low in foods such as fruits and vegetables, whole grains, and legumes, which have a good balance of both omega-6 and omega-3 essential fatty acids. By contrast, the Mediterranean diet is high in oily fish and nuts, fruits and vegetables, and legumes, all of which favor omega-3s. If this is true, then getting back to the peasant food favored in small fishing villages in the Mediterranean and on the Riviera will be just the cure we need.

What They Eat in Saint-Tropez

The diet of the typical resident or tourist in Saint-Tropez is healthy because it is based on the very first convenience foods, foods that were once the easiest to obtain and the most plentiful. This ancient and healthy diet consists of:

Fresh foods. This means fruits, colorful vegetables, herbs, and dark leafy greens in abundance. In Saint-Tropez, Tuesday and Saturday are market days. If you lived here, you would take a big basket to market where you would see, smell, and examine the freshest produce available that day. You would choose what to cook for dinner based on foods harvested that day, and you would talk to the people who grew and picked those vegetables. In Saint-Tropez, you would not think about food less. Actually, you would think about it more often. At home in the United States, you might feel hungry and then look for something quick and easy (and therefore, probably prepackaged and loaded with calories) to satisfy that urge. In Provence, you would be thinking of food and planning meals all day long, so that hunger is no surprise, and healthy food to satisfy that hunger is readily available.

When you cooked with these vegetables and fruits, you would not be constrained only to steaming or roasting vegetables. You could purée them into a sauce. You could chop greens and sauté them with herbs and wine. You would use your own instincts and creativity to construct each meal.

Plenty of fish. Saint-Tropez is a fisherman's paradise. Here you can go directly to the docks to buy freshly caught fish, or you can go to any restaurant to enjoy fresh fish in soups or salads or with interesting sauces. You might enjoy fish not commonly available in Western markets such as fresh sardines, red mullet, and whiting (all native to the Mediterranean). You would eat fish prepared in inventive ways, such as Salmon and Fennel Papilotte, Hake with Leek Fondue, Tuna with Balsamic Vinegar, or Mackerels with Mushrooms.

Smaller portions of meat. In your own kitchen, you might have come to think of dinner in fairly narrow terms, such as meat—usually chicken, pork, or beef—accompanied by a starch and a vegetable. Or if you had a really long day at work, variety might mean fast food, takeout, or pasta. That's about it. In Saint-Tropez, you would enjoy entirely new tastes and combinations of food, mostly based on fresh fish, at every meal. Sure, there would be meat, but it might be rabbit stew, quail cooked with grapes, or pork roast with figs. You would enjoy them in slightly smaller portions with bright new flavor combinations.

Nuts, seeds, and legumes. Have you ever had broccoli with pistachio dressing? Fava beans with ham or duck? How about spinach cooked with pine nuts and raisins, or white bean stew? In Saint-Tropez, chefs view nuts, seeds, and legumes as important proteins on which to build meals and layer tastes. The Western diet is stacked with protein, but it usually comes in the form of meat, which is densely caloric and loaded with saturated fat. By trying dishes rich in vegetable proteins such as nuts, seeds, and legumes, you will cut calories and saturated fat and replace them with healthy plant-based fats, which are instead loaded with important essential fatty acids. You will also discover the big flavors of nuts and seeds and the high-fiber punch of legumes such as lentils, peas, and beans.

Oils instead of butter. In Saint-Tropez, you would never be served a salad with a bottled, nonfat dressing. Instead, you would eat salads tossed with a vinaigrette made of olive, walnut, or—for special occasions—avocado oil. You would eat vegetables sautéed or roasted with olive oil. When you eat a wider variety of foods and season them with fresh herbs and new combinations of seasonings, you'll find that you need less butter, with its high saturated fat content, as a source of flavoring.

Whole grains instead of white breads. Right now, you may be used to a diet based on white bread, white rice, and white flour. You probably eat several baked goods over the course of a day, along with cereal at breakfast, a sandwich at lunch, and a healthy dose of rice or pasta at dinner. In Saint-Tropez, by contrast, you would eat much smaller amounts of these foods. Bread would be a slight accent to a meal, not the basis. And the breads you were served would contain whole grains and lots of fiber. Some also contain walnuts, sesame seeds, or other ingredients that add omega-3 essential fatty acids and other nutrients. Other whole grains you might eat include socca, a flatbread made with chickpea flour, or fava and lima beans. Even in desserts, white flour plays only a guest appearance in crêpes or pastry crust, while the dessert gains its sweetness from fruits and its richness from nuts.

A passion for food. In Saint-Tropez, no one feels guilty about eating or loving food, and no one thinks of food as a source of stress, as something that makes them fat. If you lived there, you would love to eat every day. You would learn to love cooking every day and mealtime would be a happy, communal event and a chance to relax.

Benefits of the Saint-Tropez Diet

In 2003, researchers at the University of Athens Medical School and the Harvard School of Public Health published the largest study to date on the effects of the Mediterranean diet. In this study, researchers questioned 22,000 participants throughout Greece who were aged 50 and older about their diets. These people answered a questionnaire about the foods they ate regularly. The study showed that participants who ate a diet higher in fat than the traditional American diet but richer in fruits and vegetables, fish, olive oil and canola oil, nuts, legumes, and whole grains, can expect to reduce their risk of death by heart attack by 33 percent and their risk of death from cancer by 24 percent.

Additional studies have shown a link between this type of diet, which is high in omega-3 essential fatty acids, and other important health benefits, including:

- Slower rate of aging
- Increased energy
- Greater alertness and mental clarity
- Lower blood pressure
- Decreased systemic inflammation in the skin and tissues (systemic inflammation has been linked to Alzheimer's, heart disease, and other diseases)
- Increased ability to control blood sugar among diabetics
- Decrease in depression

The newest studies indicate that eating foods naturally high in omega-3 essential fatty acids combined with foods naturally rich in vitamin A brings additional benefits, including an increase in metabolism that triggers natural weight loss.

Why Does This Diet Work?

It seems impossible that changing your diet can have all of those effects on the body, but it does.

First of all, adding omega-3 essential fatty acids to your body (in the form of foods such as flaxseed meal, salmon, and walnuts) can reverse the effects of the modern American diet, which is loaded with sugar, refined white flour, and chemicals used to create pantry products that won't spoil. The mass production of food has brought many prepackaged foods into our kitchens. Most people have pantries stocked with boxes and cans of ready-to-eat meals and ready-to-mix baked goods.

While these foods have been marketed as convenience foods, they are really the foods most convenient to produce and store. They are "shelf-stable," which means they contain additives and preservatives that keep them from spoiling. They also contain corn-based

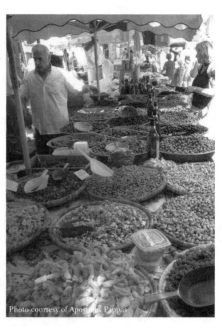

Photo courtesy of Apostolos Pappas

products, such as high fructose corn syrup and corn oil, which are easy to produce in high quantities and are loaded with empty calories. In addition, corn oil is loaded with omega-6 fatty acids.

These ingredients, the emulsifiers and preservatives, offer no nutritional content at all. Instead, a diet loaded with these processed flours, sugars, corn oil, and chemicals will clog your system, promote systemic inflammation, and advance your aging process. Above all, they are a drag on your natural metabolism. They interfere with your body's ability to store energy inside your cells and they shut down your body's system that regulates the storage of fat. All of this results in chronically low energy and greater fat deposits.

Once you balance your omega-6 and omega-3 essential fatty acid intake, your energy level will soar and your waistline will shrink.

Eat Fat, Don't Store It

For years you have been told that eating fat makes you fat. This is not true. What matters is not the quantity but the quality of the fat. Not all dietary fats are bad. In fact, your cells need omega-3 essential fatty acids in order to use and balance stored energy and communicate with each other. Study after study shows that when you starve your body of these fats, you wreak internal havoc on your body. What happens when you don't have enough omega-3s?

- Your body begins to hoard fat of every kind.
- Cells begin to miscommunicate, which gives cancerous cells the upper hand.
- Individual cells fail to use and store as much energy as they need.
- The body undergoes a crisis of inflammation, which promotes aging. Homocysteine levels increase. This is a marker for heart disease, because inflammation often takes place inside arteries.
- Your brain—which is the greatest consumer of essential fatty acids—suffers, which can lead to depression or other mental disorders.

When you have a relatively balanced diet rich in omega-3 essential fatty acids, you experience the opposite.

- Your body burns fat at a much higher rate.
- Your cells work effectively and resist corruption by cancerous toxins.
- Individual cells increase their metabolism, increasing your energy levels and maximizing your workouts.
- Systemic inflammation recedes, making you look and feel younger, and making your body more resistant to chronic illnesses.
- Your mood, and even your problem-solving ability, improves.

How Does the Saint-Tropez Diet Compare to Other Popular Diets?

Each trend in weight loss has brought a new theory on how the body burns fuel and uses fat and, thus, how best to lose weight. A few of these theories, as presented in recent books, have added greatly to our understanding of dieting and have set the stage for the Saint-Tropez Diet. These include:

The Montignac Method. Twenty years ago, nutritionist Michel Montignac was the first to introduce the concept of dieting by choosing to eat foods with a low glycemic index (GI) rather than restricting calories. These low GI foods, such as whole grains, vegetables, and certain fruits, contain fewer simple sugars and more fiber than high glycemic index foods. Therefore, they don't raise insulin levels in the blood as much as high GI foods such as white flour, sugar, and white rice. As a result, people following this diet can reduce their chances of developing type 2 diabetes and insulin resistance while they are losing weight. Montignac has written more than 20 books detailing various aspects of his diet, including the best-selling *Eat Yourself Slim* (2004) and *The French Diet* (2005). Montignac has also written books about the role of Provençal cooking in his diet, and how the French attitude toward eating and the culture of food in France has informed his methods.

The diet focuses primarily on choosing foods according to the glycemic index rather than the amount of omega-3s in any particular food. Still, Montignac has made important contributions to the theory of healthy eating by emphasizing the qualities of healthy foods outside the strict boundaries of calories and fat content.

South Beach Diet. In 2003, cardiologist Arthur Agatston unleashed his diet theory on dieters who were weary both of the low-fat diets and of high-fat/no-carbohydrate diets such as Atkins. The South Beach Diet is essentially an improved Atkins-like diet that is healthier and easier to stick to over the long term. In the initial phase, you remove starches and sugars from your diet entirely, then slowly phase them back in over time. It also introduced many dieters to the notion that there are good (unsaturated) fats, as well as bad (saturated) fats. Because it balances both a low-fat and low-carb component, this diet resembles nothing so much as the American Heart Association Diet, with a slightly more liberal view on fat. Far easier to maintain than either Atkins or the highly fat restrictive Pritkin diet often recommended to heart patients, this diet became a national sensation.

The diet in its original form contains very little discussion about essential fatty acids omega-3 and omega-6, which are the core of the Saint-Tropez Diet. Still, it does emphasize fresh fruits and vegetables, lean meats, and moderate amounts of whole grains. This book has been an important step toward changing the way Americans eat, by taking away their refined starches and replacing them with fresh, high-fiber ingredients.

The Omega Diet. In 1999, Artemis P. Simopoulos, M.D., pooled all of her research as a pioneer in the emerging field of omega-3 essential fatty acids and their effect on the human body and published this remarkable book explaining why the Mediterranean diet is so healthy. This was the first diet to detail the effects of omega-3s and their importance in overall health. It offers a great description of the various essential fatty acids and which foods contain them in the highest amounts, and it details at length the studies Simopoulos has conducted on how increasing omega-3 intake can help those with heart disease, high blood pressure, and diabetes.

Since then, books about the health benefits of omega-3s have proliferated, most focusing on the health aspects of omega-3s, while few of them detail the powerful role of essential fatty acids in weight loss. None of them have used the important research that this book presents on the effects of nutraceuticals, or health-promoting foods, particularly when consumed in combination with a diet rich in omega-3s.

The Perricone Weight-Loss Diet. This diet, published in 2005, offers an excellent description of the way that diet affects aging as well as weight. This was one of the first books to embrace and combine many of the landmark discoveries of earlier diets. Perricone urges readers to give up on sugary, processed foods and those with a high glycemic index; he extols the virtues of foods rich in omega-3 essential fatty acids (particularly salmon); and he details many so-called "superfoods," some of which are in supplement form, that Perricone says are essential to maintain good health and youthful looks.

Although much of the science surrounding good food and its relationship to overall health is sound, the notion that we all should be taking a daily regimen of high-potency supplements in order to stay healthy is controversial—and expensive. Although some scientists rigorously support the notion that supplements can and should be used to treat certain nutritional deficiencies in some individuals, many others contend that offering large numbers of people daily mega-doses of engineered vitamins and minerals is potentially toxic. In several studies, supplements appear to have no more efficacy than food products. In fact, isolated and engineered vitamins and chemicals might be utterly ignored by the body or interpreted as toxins when they don't arrive in whole foods. As scientists continue to unravel the incredible power of whole foods, they are finding that nature does a much better job of bundling vitamins, minerals, and phytochemicals for optimum health than any manufacturer.

French Women Don't Get Fat. Not so much a diet as a way of thinking about food, this book, published in 2004, preaches that moderation in all things is the key to staying thin. This concept is fundamental to French culture, which worships eating but not gluttony. Author Mirelle Guillano also details the French passion for preparing and eating food along with walking and an active lifestyle. In a way, Guillano brings dieting full circle back to the concept of fewer calories as the foundation for healthy eating—a foundation upon which the Saint-Tropez Diet builds.

Improving the Mediterranean and Provençal Diet

By conducting studies in how food combining and neutraceuticals affect the body, scientists are discovering ways to improve this natural diet, making it even healthier and more efficient at burning fat. These new studies show that omega-3 essential fatty acids work best with certain nutrients in fruits and vegetables, sometimes called phytonutrients, to boost their healthful qualities.

In the next few chapters you'll learn how essential fatty acids work with nutrients to change the way your cells function. These new discoveries are the basis for the Saint-Tropez Diet, which addresses for the first time the exciting new research about the importance of:

1. Boosting omega-3 intake
2. Combining omega-3 essential fatty acids with vitamin A
3. Reducing omega-6 intake
4. Counteracting the oxidative effect of omega-3s by consuming a wide range of antioxidants and other nutraceuticals

Together, these four steps will help you reach the right ratio of omega-6 to omega-3 essential fatty acids and nutraceuticals in your body to optimize your fat-burning potential.

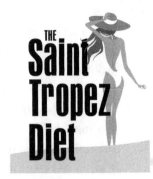

The Good and the Bad of Fat

If you have tried to lose weight in the past, you have probably found yourself buying so-called diet foods. For decades, these foods have all been labeled "low-fat." Despite the low-carbohydrate fad, most dieters still view fat as the primary gastronomic villain, and to combat it, they buy low-fat versions of foods and cook low-fat versions of their favorite cookies, cakes, and desserts. These foods are hopelessly confusing to dieters because they seem to be healthy; they seem to have cut out an inherently unhealthy aspect of a food while preserving the rest intact. By doing so, these foods encourage overeating. Why not eat 10 cookies? After all, they're low-fat!

The first thing you have to learn about changing your diet is that you are probably not eating too much fat. In fact, if you are overweight and have a pantry stocked with low-fat foods, the chances are good that your diet does not contain enough fat. More specifically, it does not contain the kinds of fats that will keep you thin and healthy.

Fat is not an evil substance. Fat is simply any substance that does not dissolve in water, and this is important because your body is made up almost entirely of water. There is fluid inside every cell in your body, and that fluid is surrounded and contained by a membrane made of fat.

About 50 percent of your brain is also made of fat, and it needs fatty acids in order to maintain its normal functions. It's true. Your brain needs fat in order to think clearly and to stave off such disorders as depression. Your body also needs fat to create hormones such as estrogen and testosterone.

Fat is so crucial to your health that your body will actually fight to protect its fat reserves by triggering hunger pangs and cravings. The average healthy woman has about 25 percent body fat. For the average man, the amount is closer to 18 percent. Any less than that and your body is likely to live in a kind of crisis mode, constantly craving the fats you deny it.

Even people who have stored quite a lot of excess fat in some obvious spots may be living in this same crisis mode. If you are overweight, your body is probably storing excess fat in part because it feels starved of the types of fats it needs most to survive. Throughout this chapter, you'll learn how to identify and eat the right kinds of fats that tell your body to shed pounds, while avoiding the types of fat that signal the need to hoard and store fat.

A diet loaded with these healthy fats is more successful because it's easier to maintain. Most people who have tried to maintain a low-fat diet have found themselves fatter and less healthy after dieting. It sounds crazy, but it's true. Most people find that a low-fat diet is notoriously difficult to stick to; when people cheat on those diets, they generally do so by making the worst possible choices because when your body is telling you that you are starving, any food seems better than none at all. Thus, the starvation-binge style of nonfat dieting generally leads to weight gain in the long term, rather than weight loss.

Types of Fats

The truth is that fats are not all alike. The fat inside a pat of butter is different from the fat in a tablespoon of olive oil, which is different from the fat in a tablespoon of margarine. Not only are they different nutritionally, they are far different substances. What's most striking about these choices is that the fats they contain don't resemble each other in the least.

- One is loaded with saturated fat, or animal fat.
- One is high in a type of unsaturated fat that comes from plants rather than animals.
- One contains a completely synthetic form of fat, known as hydrogenated fat or trans fatty acids, which is what food labels call trans fat.

Do you know which is which? Even if you don't, your body does. It reacts differently to each type of fat. Chemically, fats are composed of carbon and hydrogen atoms. Each type of fat differs in the number of atoms and the types of bonds that hold them together. Saturated fats are so-called because they are saturated with hydrogen; they already hold as many hydrogen atoms as they can, and they have no double bonds between their carbon atoms. Unsaturated fats, as we'll learn more about later in this chapter, have two main subcategories. Monounsaturated fats have one double bond in their chain of carbon atoms; polyunsaturated fats have more than one double bond. (If you're interested in learning more about different types of fatty acids, the Lipid Library website at www.lipidlibrary.co.uk is a good resource.)

In our example above, butter contains saturated fat, which is likely to be broken down into particles that will raise blood cholesterol, especially the tiny particles known as LDL (bad cholesterol). Some LDL particles may collect in your bloodstream and block your arteries, contributing to heart disease. The good news is that at least your body knows how to deal with saturated fat.

More disturbing is what the body does with hydrogenated fat, the synthetic kind that makes up many processed foods. It can hardly be called food at all. It is vegetable oil that has had hydrogen blown into it in order to make a stiff, lard-like substance that is spreadable, like margarine, or that can sit on a shelf without turning rancid, like shortening. This is the hidden health hazard in so many so-called diet foods.

Hydrogenated fat is a fake food; it has few nutritional components that would be readily understood by your digestive system. The trouble is that your body has no idea what to do with it or how to break it down. If the body processes it as saturated fat, as it usually does, then it will go directly to fatty deposits. If not, the hydrogenated fat will circulate until it (like the LDL from saturated fats) gets caught up in the plaques in your arteries, increasing your risk of heart problems. The Food and Drug Administration (FDA) recently established new guidelines requiring manufacturers to list trans fatty acids in nutrition labels. So look for trans fat (or hydrogenated or partially hydrogenated oils). But be aware that manufacturers are allowed to round down the

GIVE UP ON TRANS FATS

Giving up hydrogenated oils and the nasty trans fats that come along with them is easy to say and harder to do. You'll have to read food labels carefully to find these synthetic fats. Here are some tips.

1. *Anything that has a creamy or cheese-like consistency but that is stored at room temperature, such as in a vending machine, contains trans fat. This includes most frostings or fillings that can sit at room temperature.*
2. *Most chips, crackers, and pastries with long shelf lives are made with hydrogenated oils to make them last longer in supermarkets.*
3. *Anything that contains "partially hydrogenated" oils (even if they seem healthy, such as soybean oil) are unhealthy.*
4. *Most boxed convenience foods, including cookie and cake mixes, contain trans fats.*
5. *Foods containing butter flavorings, such as microwave popcorn, can contain high amounts of trans fats.*
6. *If the word "hydrogenated" appears anywhere on the list of ingredients, the product contains trans fat—even if the product also says "zero trans fats per serving." Remember, manufacturers can round down their estimates of certain fats. That means that if a bag of chips or cookies contains less than 0.5 grams of trans fat per serving, the manufacturer can legally claim that it contains zero trans fats per serving, while ignoring the fact that people are likely to eat more than one serving at a time.*

amount of fat declared on the nutrition label: If a food has a per serving amount that is less than 0.5 grams, it can be listed as having zero trans fat.

Of the three examples above, the healthiest is the tablespoon of olive oil, which contains unsaturated fat. Your body might store these in the same fatty deposits as saturated fats when consumed in excess.

However, because unsaturated fats are much more complex, they will more likely be used by cells to be stored as energy or to build cell walls or other structural components of the cell.

These fats combine with and bolster the health benefits of other foods. For example, tomatoes contain a substance called lycopene that has been shown to inhibit cancer cells. Studies have also shown that when tomatoes are cooked and eaten with olive oil, the lycopene is more readily absorbed by the body. Researchers have found a similar effect when vegetables high in beta carotene, the natural form of vitamin A, are eaten in combination with plant-based oils such as olive oil or walnut oil. According to these studies, full-fat salad dressings trump low-fat dressings with synthetic ingredients because they boost the nutritional value of the vegetables they are served with. They also contain unsaturated fats, the good fats, that have important health benefits of their own.

Understanding Unsaturated Fats

Although it's clear that giving up all forms of trans fats and reducing the amount of saturated fat you eat will help you lose weight and feel healthier, what about those unsaturated fats? They seem much better, and they are, but even these vary widely in their nutritional value and in how your body reacts to them. Unsaturated fats are found in certain types of foods, including oily fish such as salmon, sardines, mackerel, and trout. These fats are also found in fatty plant-based foods such as avocado, nuts, and seeds. The primary way to add unsaturated fats to your diet is through cooking oils used to sauté vegetables, added to baked goods, or mixed into salad dressing.

There are two main types of unsaturated fats: monounsaturated and polyunsaturated fats.

Monounsaturated fats, as we noted earlier, have only one double bond in their chemical structure. Monounsaturated fats usually stay liquid at room temperature in contrast to saturated fat, which is usually solid. Oleic acid, which is found in olive oil, is one of the most common types of monounsaturated fats.

Oils rich in monounsaturated fatty acids include:

Olive oil

Canola oil

Avocado oil

Grades of sunflower oil high in oleic acid

Polyunsaturated fat, with two or more double bonds in its chemical structure, is usually of vegetable origin and also usually liquid at room temperature. For decades, food scientists and nutritionists didn't make any distinction between monounsaturated and polyunsaturated fats, but this has changed in the last few decades. Now researchers know that polyunsaturated fats are far different from monounsaturated fats. Some of them contain high amounts of particular fatty acids that your body uses to regulate everything from inflammation to blood sugar levels to the amount of fat stored in your body.

Oils rich in polyunsaturated fatty acids include:

Borage oil

Fish oil

Flaxseed oil

Grapeseed oil

Peanut oil

Sesame oil

Soybean oil

Walnut oil

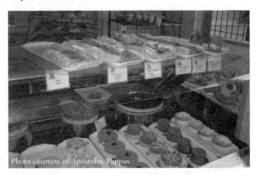
Photo courtesy of Apostolos Pappas

Yet not all polyunsaturated fats are alike. In fact, not all of them are fats that will help you lose weight. There are two main types of polyunsaturated fats, omega-3s and omega-6s; in turn, there are different types of omega-3 and omega-6 fats.

Omega-3 Essential Fatty Acids

Scientists have studied the effects of omega-3 essential fatty acids on the body for more than a decade now, and the results of this research are startling. According to Artemis P. Simopoulos, M.D., in *The Omega Diet*, omega-3s lower bad cholesterol, reduce inflammation, slow the formation of blood clots, help prevent high blood pressure and irregular heartbeat, and reduce plaque formation in our arteries.

A FAT BY ANY OTHER NAME...

As we've learned, fats are composed of carbon and hydrogen atoms. Each type of fat differs in the number of carbon and hydrogen atoms and the types of bonds that hold them together. Almost all of the fats in our diet are triglycerides—that is, they are composed of three fatty acids. For this reason, you'll often see dietary fats referred to as "fatty acids"—and, as we get a little deeper into our discussion of the different types of fats, you'll see that many types of fats are referred to simply as "acids" (such as linoleic acid or alpha-linolenic acid). You'll also see the term "essential fatty acids (EFAs)" bandied about. This refers to the fatty acids (including omega-3s and omega-6s) that our bodies cannot synthesize and that we therefore need to get from food.

Finally, as you've seen, most of our sources of dietary fat are oils, so you will sometimes see the terms "fats" and "oils" used interchangeably. Keep in mind that most oils and dietary fats are made up of more than one type of fatty acid. Canola oil, for instance, contains saturated fatty acids, monounsaturated fatty acids, and at least two types of polyunsaturated fatty acids. But because it has a greater percentage of monounsaturated fatty acids than the other types of fatty acids, you will usually see it categorized simply as a good source of monounsaturated fat. Similarly, beef, which is considered bad for you because it is high in saturated fat, also contains some unsaturated fatty acids.

Scientific studies have also shown that diets high in omega-3s lower your risk of developing cancer while reducing the growth rate of tumors and increasing the effectiveness of traditional cancer treatments. Here is a quick summary of some of these studies.

It is heart healthy. One study conducted in 2005 at Emory University led by Fernando Holguin randomly offered 58 elderly nursing home residents fish oil pills or soy oil pills and then tracked their hearth health for six months. The people given omega-3 pills had healthier heart rhythms after six months than those who did not.

It has anti-inflammatory properties. Inflammation is the basis for disease and advanced aging. Even cancer cells begin as an inflammation. So does heart disease. Omega-3 essential fatty acids help block the systemic process of inflammation. Arthritis sufferers have long used fish oil pills as a kind of over-the-counter treatment for swollen joints.

In one study conducted at Penn State University in 2004, researchers tracked the effects of three different diets: the modern American diet; a diet rich in a type of omega-3 essential fatty acid; and a diet rich in a type of omega-6 essential fatty acid. Both the omega-3 and omega-6 diets decreased total and LDL cholesterol levels, but the omega-3 diet appeared to be most effective in reducing cardiovascular disease risk, possibly by combating vascular inflammation. At the conclusion of the study, the people eating the typical American diet had the highest amount of C-reactive protein, a substance that indicates a high level of systemic inflammation and a marker for future heart disease. Of the other two groups, the people eating high amounts of omega-3 oils had the lowest amount of C-reactive protein.

It improves brain health. A couple of recent studies have shown that the children of mothers who took in high amounts of omega-3 oils during pregnancy have slightly higher IQs and fewer behavioral problems than those whose mothers consumed little or no omega-3 oils during pregnancy.

In 2005, researchers in Siena, Italy gave people a pill that either contained a fish oil supplement (which is high in omega-3 fatty acids) or an olive oil supplement (which is not) for 35 days. The aim of the study was to test whether omega-3 fatty acid supplementation would change cognitive function. At the end of the study, the people who had been consuming fish oil did far better on various tests that measured their ability to concentrate and reason. Incidentally, they were also in a much better mood than participants taking olive oil supplements. Researchers concluded that the differences between the two groups were linked to the increase in omega-3 essential fatty acids.

It promotes weight loss. Omega-3s transport fatty acids into the mitochondria of our cells for burning as fuel and also influence the body's need to store fat. In effect, they turn a master switch inside your metabolism that tells your body to burn stored fatty acids, a phenomenon we'll explore in a little more detail in chapter 4.

There are two types of omega-3 essential fatty acids most associated with health benefits, and they have rather long and complicated names. One is eicosapentaenoic acid (EPA) and the other is docosahexaenoic acid (DHA). There's no reason for you to memorize these names, but you should know that these are the most powerful forms of omega-3 essential fatty acids and that they are only found in animal fats, such as oily fish and meats taken from animals that were fed a wide variety of greens including wild grasses rather than a bland diet of corn mush.

In addition, green leafy vegetables, flaxseed, walnuts, and some other nuts and seeds contain alpha-linolenic acid (usually abbreviated LNA, although you may also see it referred to as ALA). It may be difficult to imagine that spinach, lettuce, or other green leaves contain these oils, but they do. Even though fruits and vegetables aren't oily, they do have cells—and these cells have membranes made of oils rich in fatty acids. Our bodies convert LNA to EPA, but only to a small extent, so you need to consume more LNA than EPA or DHA in order to get the same health benefits. LNA is still tremendously healthful, though, and is the only source of omega-3s for vegetarians.

There are a host of products now available in supermarkets and health food stores that claim to boost your essential fatty acids and increase your omega-3 intake. These include sports drinks, weight loss bars, and fish oil pills. While these may be rich in of omega-3 essential fatty acids, the most effiecient and least expensive sources are those that come from nature's own foods.

To increase your intake of omega-3 essential fatty acids, eat:

- Fish, particularly oily coldwater fish, such as salmon, tuna, sardines, herring, mackerel, anchovies (you can soak them in water for 15 minutes to remove some of the salt), trout, and bluefish. It's best to steam, bake, or broil your fish, since frying destroys the healthy oils. Ideally, you would be taking in 2 to 3 servings per week.
- Nuts and seeds, primarily walnuts and ground flaxseed;

secondarily, pine nuts, butternuts, and pumpkin seeds. You should be taking in a few tablespoons per day of nuts and seeds rich in these fatty acids.

- Grass-fed meats, including free-range poultry, beef, lamb, and other lean meats. The eggs of poultry fed greens that contain omega-3s are also going to have higher amounts of beneficial fat. Plan to eat 2 to 3 servings per week.

- Fruits and vegetables, especially dark leafy greens. All fruits and vegetables contain trace amounts of omega-3s, but more importantly, they have the right ratio of omega-3 to omega-6 oils. The more you consume of these healthy foods, the more likely you are to regain a healthy balance of fatty acids in your body. Plan to eat 5 servings or more each day.

Some nutritionists are so high on the health benefits and anti-aging benefits of omega-3 essential fatty acids that they actually recommend taking fish oil pills several times a day in order to gain what they claim are the best results. But in reality, no studies have yet confirmed that these extremely high doses of omega-3s have any additional benefits over what can be consumed by eating whole foods in a normal, healthy diet. We simply don't know yet what the exact optimal level of omega-3 consumption is, although recent studies—and the traditional Mediterranean diet—suggest that about 1 gram per day is healthy provided omega-6 consumption is no more than 4 grams. If you eat 8 grams of omega-6s, increase omega-3s to 2 to 3 grams. Remember, the ratio of omega-6 to omega-3 essential fatty acids is important.

And while we don't yet know of any adverse side effects from taking too-high doses of omega-3 supplements, consider the history of vitamin supplements. Eating foods rich in vitamins is healthy. And yet there are many adverse side effects, such as stomach upset or in rare cases kidney stones and liver toxicity, that come from overloading on vitamin supplements and fortified foods such as energy bars and energy drinks. The same rationale, in my opinion, applies to the omega-3s. Like vitamins, we do not synthesize them but use them for normal physiological functions. So stick to whole foods as your source of omega-3s; they're safer as well as tastier.

In addition, omega-3 pills can be quite expensive, between 10 cents to 30 cents per pill, so taking three or more per day can add up to a fairly significant annual bill. Few companies actually produce omega-3 pills because it is a substance that is hard to synthesize. The oil has to be pressed from plant seeds, nuts, grains, and fish, which is an expensive process.

Also, although the pills themselves may claim to have 1,000 milligrams of omega-3s, the ones produced from plant seed oils contain far smaller amounts of the healthy fatty acids, DHA and EPA, so the health-boosting elements of these pills may be far smaller than advertised. So if you do take supplements, look for ones made from fish oils. These contain far more EPA and DHA oils, which are more efficiently absorbed into your cells and are thus more likely to give you the benefits you're looking for.

Gorging yourself on foods rich in omega-3s will not give you any additional benefits, either. Even if you wanted to boost your omega-3s by eating three pounds of salmon per day, for example, that would not necessarily translate into greater health benefits. Everything is best consumed in moderation.

The most important thing to remember is that you do not need to eat a lot of omega-3 essential fatty acids to gain all of their advantages on your health and your waistline. If you follow the Saint-Tropez Diet, you will consume all the omega-3 essential fatty acids you need.

Omega-6 Essential Fatty Acids

Currently, the standard American diet favors highly processed wheat products, white rice, and pasta, all of which contain lots of starch. It also emphasizes proteins, primarily derived from meats raised on farms where they are fed a steady and bland diet of corn products, which are very high in omega-6 essential fatty acids. Our diet also tends to favor highly processed vending machine foods and boxed convenience foods that are created specifically for their ability to withstand spoilage for months at a time, rather than their ability to nourish the body. Not surprisingly, these products are also high in omega-6 essential fatty acids.

The American diet is loaded with these omega-6s, which are primarily found in:

- Refined grains
- Most vegetable oils
- Meats from animals that are not grass-fed
- Baked goods

Some researchers estimate that the amount of omega-6 essential fatty acids consumed in the American diet has doubled in the past 40 years, in part because of the increase in shelf-stable baked goods in our diet along with the increase in the use of corn oil, shortening, and other vegetable oils rich in omega-6 (such as sunflower, soybean, and cottonseed) for baking and frying foods.

As a result, scientists announced at the 2004 meeting of the International Society for the Study of Fatty Acids and Lipids that many of the diseases so common today are potentially the results of omega-6 overconsumption, which also has obesity as a side effect. Many chronic diseases, from arthritis to heart disease to cancer, are characterized by an overproduction of pro-inflammatory molecules, for which omega-6 essential fatty acids are precursors. Omega-6s also often lower HDL (good cholesterol) levels and increase the oxidation of LDL (bad cholesterol), which also has an inflammatory effect.

Gorging on omega-6s exclusively while ignoring omega-3s correlates with the increased incidence of many diseases, such as cancer, depression, macular degeneration, and heart disease. In animal experiments, diets rich in omega-6 essential fatty acids increased the body weight to a much higher degree than diets with equal amounts of omega-3 essential fatty acids. Righting this balance in your diet will have powerful long-term effects on your health in addition to keeping you thin.

So, while you are increasing your intake of omega-3 essential fatty acids, you will want to minimize the effects of the modern diet by taking in fewer omega-6 essential fatty acids. To do that, you should:

- Avoid vegetable oils that have a poor ratio of omega-6 to omega-3 oils. These include corn, safflower, sunflower, cottonseed, soybean, borage, sesame, and peanut oil, which are often found in highly processed foods.

THE BENEFITS OF OLIVE OIL

Although olive oil does not have a particular concentration of omega-3 essential fatty acids, it is a good, healthy fat to consume regularly. Olive oil contains oleic acid, the most predominant fatty acid in all of the tissues of your body. When your body is low on oleic acid, your body tries to synthesize it because it is an essential part of our metabolism. This causes your body to hoard and store fat in an effort to keep supplies available. By eating olive oil regularly, you give your body a ready supply of oleic acid and tell your body that it does not need to hoard fat.

Olive oil also contains in small quantities many molecules with antioxidant activities such as vitamin E and squalene, which also lower cholesterol.

Also, olive oil is resistant to high heat. Many oils, such as corn oil and safflower oil, have a relatively low smoke point (the point at which they will start to smoke when exposed to high heat). Once oils have been exposed to moderate heat, they oxidize, thereby losing their beneficial qualities and developing offensive odors. Olive oil is resistant to this change and therefore can be used safely as a coating for roasted and sautéed vegetables without losing its beneficial profile.

Although most food labels don't list fatty acid components of oils and foods, these labels will sometimes list the presence of oleic acid. Look for the mention of oleic acid or monounsaturates in these foods.

- Avoid highly processed foods, especially those that contain refined flours, such as white bread, or highly refined grains, such as white rice.
- Buy foods that contain omega-3s instead.

Keep in mind, however, that omega-6s are still essential fatty acids—that is, they are essential to your health and well-being. Omega-6s help regulate your metabolism and maintain skin health, among other benefits. So you still need them in your diet; you just need fewer of them than you are probably consuming now.

Conjugated Linoleic Acid

A lot has been written about the effects of this particular fatty acid both on general health and on weight loss. Conjugated linoleic acid is a type of fatty acid found exclusively in milk and meat products, where its presence challenges the notion that red meat and whole milk are by their nature unhealthy. In fact, CLA has been shown to have strong anti-cancer properties even in small amounts, and to decrease the rate at which glucose is transformed into fat by the body. It may enhance insulin sensitivity and therefore help the body to better regulate blood sugar levels.

Decades ago, when cattle were allowed to graze on grasses in a moderately open range, the meat we ate had a much higher level of natural CLA than it does now. These days steers and dairy cows are fed a diet of hybrid grains designed specifically to fatten them or enhance their milk production. As a result, the natural CLA in milk and meat products is far lower than it was 50 years ago.

Using this information, a few manufacturers are selling supplemental CLA derived from safflower oil as a diet aid or metabolism boost. Some early studies show that these supplements seem to be safe in moderate doses up to 3 grams per day. In one study published in the *American Journal of Clinical Nutrition* in 2004, healthy overweight adults took 4½ grams of synthetic CLA every day for one year and reduced their body weight by as much as 9 percent.[6] In a follow-up continuation of the study, the supplementation still seemed safe a year later.

Even though these supplements seem safe, it is still important to treat them with caution. Some manufacturers seem to feel that synthetic CLA is safe in extremely high doses, meaning 9 and 10 grams per day, which has not been proven in any study. In fact, no study has confirmed any actual dose as an optimum level at which to ingest this substance. It is entirely possible, and even probable, that dietary forms of CLA are sufficient for your body. An occasional glass of whole milk or full fat organic yogurt or a small portion of grass-fed beef may be all you need to keep CLA levels optimal in your body to take advantage of its weight loss and cancer-fighting properties.

The Right Fat Profile

To summarize, there are many different types of dietary fat, some of which are healthy, some very unhealthy. Here's a quick review of what you want to remember about fats:

TYPE OF FAT	HOW MUCH SHOULD YOU EAT	SOURCES
Hydrogenated/Trans	None	Margarine
Saturated	Sparingly	Butter
Unsaturated		
Monounsaturated	Primarily for cooking and salads	Olive, canola, avocado oil
Polyunsaturated		
Omega-3 (including EPA, DHA, LNA)	Every day	Oily fish, nuts, seeds, grass-fed meat, leafy dark greens
Omega-6	Reduce but don't eliminate	Corn, sunflower, soybean oil, store-bought salad dressing, convenience foods
CLA	Periodically	Milk, dairy

You already know that saturated and trans fatty acids are bad for you, and unsaturated fats are mostly good. But it's also important to keep in mind the ratio between two key types of polyunsaturated fats—omega-6 and omega-3 essential fatty acids. We don't know the precise ratio that's optimal for health and weight loss, but if you aim for a ratio of about 4 omega-6s to every omega-3, you'll be in the right range to reap the benefits of the Saint-Tropez Diet.

THE Saint Tropez Diet

Turbocharging Your Fat-Burning Receptors

For 30 years, dieters have been told to cut the fat out of their diets in order to reduce the fat in their bodies. The logic seemed simple, but now we know it was incorrect. As we've seen, you actually need to eat more of a certain kind of fat—the omega-3 essential fatty acids—in order to trim your waistline and improve your health. Why does this work? The answer is not so simple but is worth investigating. In order to figure this out, you'll want to understand how the key to your metabolism lies in each individual cell in your body.

The Human Cell

The cell is the most basic unit of life. Your body contains trillions of them, each with a designated and specific function. Your cells function as part of a group or organ, which means that they have to communicate with each other.

All cells take in nutrients, store energy, spend energy, and dispose of waste products. The mastermind of any cell is its nucleus, which contains the DNA or genetic code of the cell, telling it how to behave. All cells also have a skin, called the membrane, which protects it.

The membrane of each cell has small antennae, called receptors. There are many types of receptors, and their function is to receive messages from outside the cell. Usually these messages are carried by the molecules that we call hormones. A hormone is a chemical messenger from one cell (or group of cells) to another. Hormones can stimulate or inhibit cell growth, among other things, and are responsible for regulating metabolism. Most hormones are released directly into the bloodstream, and move by circulation or diffusion to target cells via their receptors. Therefore your cell receptors and your hormones (and other messengers) work together to determine how you will respond to stress and utilize nutrients, among other things.

Regulating Metabolism

Your metabolism is the process by which your body breaks down food into energy and other substances necessary for survival. Your basal metabolic rate is the amount of energy you burn while at rest. People with a higher metabolism burn more calories while at rest and therefore tend to gain weight more slowly. Exercise affects metabolism or the burning of energy for several hours after a workout, which is why exercise is said to boost the metabolism. A starvation diet, by contrast, will slow your metabolism because the body will sense a shortage of food and begin to conserve energy while at rest.

A diet high in omega-6 fatty acids encourages the body to store fat rather than spending it as energy, meaning that your body will burn less energy while at rest. In order to lose weight, you'll want your body to freely burn fat and energy. Increasing your omega-3 intake will do just that.

Omega-3s and Peroxisome Proliferator-Activated Receptors (PPARs)

One class of cell receptors are the peroxisome proliferator-activated receptors (PPARs). These receptors, located in the nucleus of the cell, are looking for messages not from hormones but instead directly from the nutrients you consume. Your liver and fat cells especially, require a constant stream of information from these nutrients to determine when to burn fat and when to store it.

There are three main types of PPARs.

- **Alpha:** Found mostly in liver, kidney, heart, muscle, and tissues with high metabolic rates and activity, alpha PPARs burn fat and are primarily activated by omega-3 essential fatty acids and CLA.
- **Gamma:** Found in different types of cells, but primarily in fat

cells, gamma PPARs usually store fat and are primarily activated by omega-6 essential fatty acids and their metabolites.

- **Delta** (also sometimes called **beta**): Found in almost all tissues but markedly in the brain, adipose (or fatty) tissue, and
skin, delta PPARs also burn fat—usually the stored fat in
cells. Scientists have not yet determined which type of fat is
primarily responsible for activating delta PPARs.

As noted, scientists have discovered
that omega-3 essential fatty acids
speak most powerfully to alpha
PPARs. Omega-3 essential fatty acids
bind to these receptors. Let's call
them fat-burning receptors. As such,
the fatty acids are allowed to enter the
cell and communicate directly with its
nucleus. In fact, they bond with the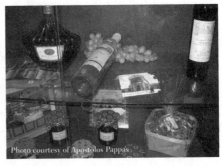
DNA inside the cell, change the cell's metabolism, and alter the way
that it uses proteins.

Omega-3 essential fatty acids stimulate the breakdown of stored
fat to energy. It's as if they tapped out a Morse code to each cell's
DNA, which then translates that code into a message that the cell un-
derstands and obeys. The message is this: Burn fat. So, when you eat
a piece of salmon or a handful of walnuts, or any food with a high concentration of omega-3s, you are sending a message directly to your
liver cells, telling them to burn fat. Eating more omega-3 essential
fatty acids is a way of reaching inside your cells and flipping a switch
that tells them to burn fat. This increases your metabolism. You will
have more energy available to you all day, and you will burn fat even
while at rest. Omega-3s work via PPARs together with retinoic acid, a
metabolite of vitamin A. As we'll learn, the omega-3s cannot work
without retinoic acid.

By contrast, omega-6 essential fatty acids or their metabolites ac-
tivate gamma PPARs, which stimulate the increase in size of fat cells
and control sugar levels in the bloodstream through a complex net-
work of signals. These receptors are most likely stimulated by linoleic

acid and other forms of omega-6 essential fatty acids (such as the proinflammatory metabolites of arachidonic acid) released when you eat junk food, fried food, and processed foods that are high in omega-6s and saturated fat. By cutting down on your intake of omega-6 essential fatty acids and increasing your intake of omega-3s, you can avoid stimulating the receptors in your cells that actually cause your body to store extra fat. So junk food makes you fat in two ways: first by adding lots of densely packed empty calories to your system, and second by telling your body to store as many calories as possible in fatty deposits.

Why do the essential fatty acids create such a powerful reaction inside your cells? Scientists aren't sure, but omega-3s were always abundant in the diet of the primitive man: fish, nuts, wild game, and leafy green vegetables. And while our diets have changed dramatically in the past 50 years, our receptors themselves have not. Quite simply, if you want to communicate directly to the cells in your body and ask them to change the way they store fat, and coincidentally, to ask them to function in a healthier and more efficient manner, you have to use the language they understand, and that language is made up of omega-3 essential fatty acids.

Because the PPARs are a direct line of communication to the DNA in your cells, they are an enormous force for nutritional good or, conversely, can wreak real incremental damage on your entire system while under the influence of junk food or refined foods high in omega-6 but low in omega-3 essential fatty acids.

PPARs can control the creation and stimulate the burning of fatty deposits, the amount of sugar in your bloodstream, and the amount of energy stored in muscle tissue. They can also control the amount of fat in your bloodstream, which is a primary pathway for developing heart disease or defects in lipid metabolism. They also help regulate inflammation throughout the system, which is a cause for heart disease and premature aging.

Other Fuels Matter, Too

Of course, essential fatty acids aren't the only forms of nutrients that can affect cells. Carbohydrates, other fats, proteins, water, vitamins and minerals are also important tools needed by cells in order for them to

PPAR-RELATED DRUGS

PPARs are so powerful at regulating the body's use of sugar and fat that scientists are trying to find a way to create a group of drugs that will have the same effect. If they are successful, they will help patients control their obesity and protect against heart disease more quickly than they could by changing their diets and adding exercise to their lives.

Unfortunately, many of the drugs currently under development have been linked to an increased incidence of cancer in mice. In response, the FDA has increased regulations covering the human testing of these drugs, and a few drug companies have abandoned these experimental drugs altogether.

Even if these drugs are introduced in the near future, they may only be prescribed to people who have established chronic conditions that require intervention, such as diabetes and heart disease. Also, they are likely to have some as yet unforeseen side effects. By contrast, the healthy diet prescribed here will have many similar effects of regulating glucose levels and reducing fat, with no side effects at all—except an increase in overall energy. And, as we've emphasized all along, the freshness and wholesomeness of the foods in your diet will go a long way toward helping you lose weight—and enjoy the process!

Just as vitamin supplements may have adverse side effects but vitamins from food do not, PPAR activators may have adverse side effects if taken as drugs or pills but are safe and healthy if eaten in their natural state, as omega-3s in foods. Nature has wisely formulated biochemically important molecules like omega-3s and vitamin A into effective (and delicious!) packages, such as fruits, vegetables, and fish. The Saint-Tropez Diet goes one step further in putting these foods together into even more effective combinations.

function properly and repair or replicate themselves. These substances work in conjunction with essential fatty acids to communicate to your cells and to help them to function efficiently and well. Eating a varied diet of healthy foods keeps your cells working efficiently and well. Exercise is also essential to keep your metabolism humming. And when your body is working at its peak, your stamina in your workouts will increase, which will also increase your ability to lose weight and remain fit.

One of the most important of these substances is vitamin A. Dietary sources of vitamin A, including carrots, red bell peppers, mangoes, pumpkin, and other colored vegetables, help stimulate the PPARs. The body uses dietary forms of vitamin A to manufacture another chemical, called retinoic acid, and this helps the PPARs to function. Someone who consumes little or no dietary vitamin A can not benefit from the consumption of omega-3s. This could prevent your body from benefiting from other nutrients in your diet and even from burning fat.

Health Benefits of Stimulating PPARs

As we mentioned earlier, PPARs can be a powerful force for health if we stimulate the correct ones with the correct nutrients. Here are some of the many benefits of stimulating PPARs:

Reducing obesity. As we discussed above, when we eat omega-3s with sufficient amounts of vitamin A, we stimulate alpha (and maybe also delta) PPARs to burn fat. At the same time, if we avoid eating excess amounts of omega-6s, we can avoid stimulating gamma PPARs to store fat. Combined with other nutrients and with exercise, this can help us lose weight and therefore reduce obesity.

Reducing inflammation. PPAR activities are thought to inhibit inflammation throughout the body, even in inflammatory diseases, such as arthritis. Because systemic inflammation inside the arteries is considered to be a marker for heart disease, reducing that inflammation throughout the body should have a positive influence on your blood flow.

Reducing heart disease. Doctors have long prescribed a class of drugs called fibrates to people with high levels of blood triglycerides and cholesterol. These drugs are also known as PPAR-alpha agonists, which means they stimulate the same receptors that you can stimulate with a good diet high in omega-3s. Specifically, these drugs are supposed to stimulate the body's drive to burn fat and release energy, rather than allowing it to circulate in the bloodstream until it is stored or attaches itself to the arterial walls. Unfortunately, they have several side effects, some as mild as stomach upset. More rarely, they can cause kidney failure or systemic toxicity. Stimulating these receptors through a good diet has none of these side effects, but can have many of the same benefits of lowered cholesterol levels, particularly a lower LDL.

Protecting against cancer. The careful balance of cell growth and death is kept in check also by the activity of PPARs. When PPAR function is upset, this balance can be upset. It makes sense that any part of the cell that is involved in taking in nutrients and communicating with the nucleus of the cell can have a powerful influence on corrupting the DNA inside the cell. It may even communicate that corruption to neighboring cells. By contrast, there is evidence that some of these same receptors can suppress the growth of certain types of cancerous cells. Scientists are experimenting with drugs that would stimulate or suppress the relevant receptors in a way to aid traditional cancer therapies.

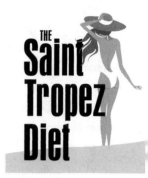

The Power of Nutraceuticals

If you have tried to eat a healthier diet in the past, you may have trained yourself to view foods in terms of their vitamin and mineral profile. Looking at a banana, you might think of its potassium. A piece of spinach might represent iron, while a carrot or red bell pepper represents vitamin A. These notions aren't incorrect, but fruits and vegetables are far more complex than just their vitamin and mineral contents.

Plant-based foods—meaning fruits, vegetables, and whole grains—contain complex chemicals. Some of these are vitamins or minerals or fatty acids that feed your cells or have a particular interaction on the individual cells in your body and may alter your DNA to prevent or treat disease or to increase your body's ability to burn fat. Other substances can also have powerful effects inside your cells.

For example, apples contain vitamin C, but researchers have recently studied apples and found that their primary healthful effect on the human body doesn't come from the vitamin C, but rather from other chemicals in the flesh and skin of the apple, often called phytochemicals, which have anti-cancer properties. Other examples include the flavonoids in blueberries, the polyphenols in red wine, and the lycopene in tomatoes. When a food is considered to have a beneficial effect on the body, it is sometimes called a functional food. Others may use a different term—nutraceutical—that is gaining popularity now. The word nutraceutical is coined from two words "nutrient" and "pharmaceutical," and it refers to the assumed medical benefits that come from certain foods.

Numerous studies have shown that eating a regular diet of fruits and vegetables will reduce your risk of developing cancer, heart disease, stroke, cataracts, and accelerated aging, but not only because they contain vitamins and minerals. Rather, it is because they contain these bioactive components that are beginning to be studied by scientists. When these substances are better understood, you may be able to eat your way back to good health. Targeted nutrition may be found to be the best way to prevent, or even treat, certain illnesses. As Hippocrates, the father of medicine, once said, "Let your food be your medicine and let your medicine be your food."

Types of Bioactive Ingredients

There are thousands of phytochemicals in foods. Here we will talk about just the most important of these chemicals for the Saint-Tropez Diet and what is thought to be their health benefits. Ongoing research will further clarify their roles in maintaining optimal health. Most of them have antioxidant activity, which reduces damage to cells from the excess of oxidation from processes such as the burning of fat. The major classes of antioxidants are:

1. **Vitamins.** Certain vitamins, such as vitamin E, vitamin C, and beta-carotene, have long been known to act as antioxidants inside the body, meaning that they work against the natural forces of oxidation inside the body. The cells inside your body are constantly exposed to oxidants, or stressors, as they perform their functions. As they do, some of the molecules inside your body lose an electron. This changes them into something called a free radical, which is toxic to your cells. To fight these free radicals and the damage they can cause, your body needs antioxidants to restore equilibrium and neutralize free radicals, thus preventing them from making cells vulnerable to mutation and disease. Although your body does manufacture its own antioxidants, it depends highly on the antioxidants coming from the diet to combat these free radicals.

2. **Polyphenols.** Found in tea, nuts, and berries, polyphenols have anti-inflammatory and anti-allergenic properties.

3. **Flavonoids.** Found in berries, herbs, vegetables, tea, and red wine, flavonoids may fight allergies, inflammation, and cancer and protect against oxidation inside the body.

4. **Cartenoids.** Found in red and yellow vegetables, caretenoids include beta-carotene, alpha-carotein, lutein, astaxanthin, zeaxanthin, and lycopene. They help protect against cancer and the effects of aging.

5. **Phytoestrogens.** Found in soy, whole wheat, and beans, these are literally plant estrogens. They act as antioxidants and may guard against prostate and breast cancer and reduce cholesterol levels.

While fruits and vegetables contain relatively small amounts of vitamin antioxidants, they contain large amounts of phytochemicals that also act as antioxidants. They can counteract the burning of fat, stimulate the immune system, affect the expression of genes inside individual cells and, regulate hormones as well as the reproduction of individual cells. They also have antibacterial and antiviral properties.

Miracle Foods

There are certain foods and families of foods that contain higher amounts of beneficial phytochemicals. Some nutritionists refer to these as super foods or miracle foods because they have so many health benefits.

Beans. A good source of lean protein and high fiber, beans also contain relatively high amounts of polyphenols, particularly beans of various colors, meaning black, yellow, and red.

Berries. These contain high amounts of flavonoids. Many contain a phytochemical called anthocyanin that works to help the body make use of vitamin C. The darker the berry, the more of this it contains. It can help reduce the effects of aging, particularly in the brain. It is also a highly powerful anti-inflammatory and antioxidant inside the body's tissues. The antioxidants inside the skins of blueberries and grapes help lower cholesterol levels. This group includes grapes, cranberries, and currants as well as fresh berries.

Cruciferous vegetables. Broccoli, Brussels sprouts, cabbage, kale, turnips, cauliflower, collards, mustard greens, and Swiss chard are some of the most powerful cancer-fighting vegetables. The phyto-chemicals inside broccoli and its cousins actually attack cancerous cells while increasing the enzymes that cleanse the body of carcinogens. They are also powerful antioxidants, particularly for the retina of the eye. If you don't like the taste of broccoli, try broccoli sprouts, which are milder in 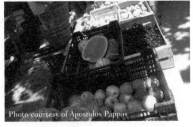 flavor but contain all of the antioxidant power of the full-grown plant.

Photo courtesy of Apostolos Pappas

Whole grains. This group includes oats, wheat germ, flaxseed, barley, spelt, couscous, brown rice, yellow corn, rye, buckwheat, and any other whole grain you can find in a health food store. Scientists are still discovering what the phytochemicals in whole grains do inside the body. Early studies suggest that these grains contain antioxidants such as vitamin B5, different forms of vitamin E, lignans, and minerals, that fight cancer and reduce the oxidative stress inside the body that contributes to aging and disease.

Wheat germ. While technically a whole grain, wheat germ has a special place in the diet because, unlike the refined grains in most flours and convenience foods, wheat germ still contains the nutrient-rich center of the wheat berry. It contains high amounts of plant-based omega-3 essential fatty acids and helps the body reduce cholesterol levels.

Flaxseed. When ground, these seeds are an important source of plant-based omega-3 essential fatty acids. They also contain phytoestrogens that help fight breast cancer.

Citrus. The most popular form of citrus must be oranges, but this group also includes lemons, limes, grapefruits, tangerines, and kumquats. More than a decade of research has linked citrus, particularly the pulp and peel, with reduced rates of cancer. Studies have shown that chemicals unique to the citrus family actually fight cell mutation that can lead to the formation of cancerous tumors.

Orange-colored foods. Most people know about carrots, but this group also includes acorn squash, butternut squash, sweet potato, red and orange bell pepper, pumpkin, cantaloupe, apricot, and mango. These fruits and vegetables contain carotenoids that protect the skin and eyes from sun damage. They also fight oxidation and cancer and stimulate the immune system.

Tomatoes. Most people are aware that tomatoes are a good source of the compound called lycopene. This is the substance that contributes to the red color of tomatoes and is available in every tomato-related product. Dietary lycopene is available in all tomato products, even processed tomatoes, such as tomato paste, purées, and tomato juice. Remember that lycopene is best absorbed by your body when cooking and you eat olive oil or some other healthy fats in the same meal.

> ### GOOD NEWS FOR THE BON VIVANTS AND BOHEMIANS
>
> *Epicatechin is a potent flavonoid that improves blood flow and therefore improves cardiac health. It is found in high amounts in dark cocoa products such as dark chocolate. Do not feel guilty anymore when you savor a piece of dark chocolate or drink some dark cocoa. Dark chocolate has been found to have nearly twice the antioxidant content of red wine and up to three times that of green tea.*

Soy. Soy is often consumed in the form of tofu, as edamame, and as soymilk or products made from soymilk. All soy products contain high amounts of phytoestrogens, known to regulate the body's levels of estrogen and help protect against hormone-related cancers such as prostate cancer and breast cancer. It also lowers cholesterol. Since there is hormonal activity, soy consumption needs to be moderate.

Dark leafy greens. These include spinach, kale, collards, bok choy, any dark-leaf lettuce, mustard greens, and turnip greens. These contain lots of carotenoids, vitamin K, chlorophyll, and some omega-3 essential fatty acids. They also contain several chemicals that lower homocysteine levels and fight sun damage in the skin. Homocysteine is an amino acid found and measured in the blood. Because high homocysteine levels have been connected to higher incidences of heart disease and stroke, some doctors suggest lowering your homocysteine levels to promote good health. The general rule is that the darker the greens the more beneficial they are.

Tea. Black and green teas are both made from the dried leaves of a particular shrub rich in neutraceuticals. Brewed tea contains thousands of healthy chemical compounds. Some of the most beneficial include flavonoids, the same substance found in grape and blueberry skins. A cup of tea also contains phytochemicals called catechins, which are highly potent antioxidants.

Nuts and seeds. The healthiest are walnuts, almonds, hazelnuts, sesame seeds, peanuts, and pumpkin seeds. They contain high amounts of polyunsaturated fatty acids (including omega-3s) and concentrated vitamins, especially E and polyphenols. Regular consumption of nuts reduces your risk of developing cancer, diabetes, and heart disease.

Allium family. Garlic, onion, scallion, leek, and other vegetables in the allium family have cancer-fighting properties and lower your LDL and homocysteine levels, thus reducing your risk for heart disease.

Herbs. Many herbs are rich in antioxidant and antibacterial chemicals and boost your immune system. Research so far has shown basil, oregano, and parsley to be highest in antioxidants.

Whole Foods Versus Supplements

While one group of scientists was studying the effects of phytochemicals from apples on the human body, and specifically on cancer cells, another group was looking at the effects of high doses of antioxidant vitamins on human cells. In this study, volunteers were given a vitamin C supplement. Afterward, their cells were tested for oxidative stress, the normal effects of aging. The people who were given this relatively high dose of what's thought to be a benign vitamin supplement showed more oxidative stress in their bodies than those who didn't take the supplement. This is a puzzling result that at least suggests that high doses of a single isolated compound might do more harm on the body than good.

Right now food manufacturers are looking for ways to isolate these healthy chemicals in order to add them to convenience foods to make them more "healthy." For example, lutein, which is found in spinach and kale, is a type of cartenoid phytochemical that may be good for your eyes. Some studies have indicated that this chemical helps reduce the chances of developing cataracts or macular eye degeneration, something many people are concerned about. Lutein helps protect against oxidative damage in the eyes. A couple of recent studies have suggested that a lutein supplement may ease the symptoms of people in the earliest stages of macular degeneration.

Already, several companies have developed lutein supplements, and one company is working on introducing a supplement that can easily be added to sports drinks, cereal bars and all sorts of baked goods. This can seem like a great idea, and may be beneficial for those at high risk of eye disease or those who have a deficiency in lutein that may have long-term consequences for their health.

But does a synthetic chemical have the power of a whole food? Does a single, isolated substance pulled from a food have the same nutritive value of that food? Is it better to consume a varied diet of whole foods or to isolate those compounds you wish to consume in greater amounts for their purported health benefits?

Given the fact that simple, water-soluble vitamin C may do some damage to the body when taken in quantities far greater than those found in nature, what could be the result of taking highly concentrated doses of these powerful nutraceuticals? The answer, of course, is that we don't really know. We do know that these powerful compounds are found in relatively small amounts in plants, sometimes in trace amounts. We suspect that they work in concert with other chemicals, many of which are as yet unidentified, to have their effects. Some clinical trials have even suggested that these chemicals have no effect on the body when taken in isolation, or at least that they have no predictable effect. The act of isolating these substances may rob them of their power to heal. In addition, no single antioxidant can replace the combination of natural healthy chemicals in whole foods.

TOXICITY OF CERTAIN VITAMINS

According to the United States Department of Agriculture (USDA), certain vitamins are toxic when taken in extremely high doses. That's why most nutritionists recommend limiting the number of fortified foods you eat in one day if you also consume a multi-vitamin. By contrast, there is no known toxicity from these same vitamins when consumed in their natural form from whole foods. For example, it is easy to take in too much vitamin A through supplements and suffer serious, if temporary, health consequences. But it is nearly impossible to eat so many carrots that you would suffer a similar toxicity. In fact, if you ate enough carrots to turn your skin orange, you still would not suffer from vitamin A toxicity. However, as always, we do suggest moderation.

Do not forget that nutraceuticals are found in foods in small doses and are biologically active in low concentrations. The biochemically important molecules are wisely formulated by nature to be safe and effective. That is why it is so important to stick to the fresh and wholesome foods that characterize the French and Mediterranean culture and form the centerpiece of the Saint-Tropez Diet.

The same may be true for omega-3 essential fatty acids and other nutraceuticals. Because the safe doses of these substances is not yet known, you should be wary when consuming these in supplement form. These supplements may result in unintended side effects.

It's clear that the antioxidant effects of fruits and vegetables far outweighs the possible benefits of any single chemical in them. In fact, different vegetables or fruits combined in a single meal or over the course of a single day may actually work together to increase the antioxidant effects of each individual food.

When you are choosing the foods in your daily diet, remember that nature is the best formulator of vitamins, minerals, and antioxidant substances. Choosing fresh fruits and vegetables along with nuts and nut oils that are high in omega-3 essential fatty acids as well as vitamin A and vitamin E will give you more antioxidant benefit than any vitamin pill or supplement.

Can You Have Too Many Nutraceuticals?

There are currently no recommended daily allowances set for any nutraceuticals, which means that relatively little is known about how much can safely be consumed before any substance becomes toxic or begins to have a negative effect. This is the primary drawback in consuming multiple nutritional supplements, particularly when there are so many bars, shakes, and sports drinks available that have also have been fortified with one or more of these chemicals. Together, these pills and shakes may have unintended consequences inside your body. Most of them have been created without having been tested on humans.

By contrast, if you are eating a wide variety of whole foods you will never be able to consume enough of these antioxidants to make yourself sick. Eating too many vitamin pills containing high doses of vitamin A can have several adverse effects, including headaches, vomiting, and peeling skin, but eating too many carrots will not. Carotene, the substance inside carrots from which the body creates vitamin A, will simply turn the skin a yellowish hue if it builds up in the system.

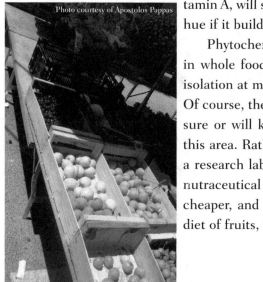
Photo courtesy of Apostolos Pappas

Phytochemicals exist in varying amounts in whole foods. These compounds taken in isolation at much higher doses may be toxic. Of course, they might not. No one knows for sure or will know until research is done in this area. Rather than use your own body as a research lab for excess use of vitamin and nutraceutical supplements, it is easier, cheaper, and healthier to consume a varied diet of fruits, vegetables, and whole grains.

The Role of Nutraceuticals in Weight Loss

At this point, you may be wondering if these nutraceuticals and the antioxidants they bring to your system actually help you lose weight. The answer is no. Aside from the fact that dramatically increasing the amount of fiber-rich foods into your diet will aid you in eating fewer calories while feeling more full, these healthy fruits and vegetables will not make your body shed weight. What they do instead is far more critical to the success of this diet.

When you increase your omega-3 intake, you are encouraging your body to burn fat. When you burn more fat, you are increasing products of oxidation, including free radicals, your system. These toxins can have a negative effect on your mood, your energy level, and even your skin tone. In fact, in the past when you tried to diet and found some success, you may have felt a little under the weather, a little worn-down, which can make diet maintenance difficult. By eating these nutrient- and antioxidant-rich foods, you will be counteracting the natural oxidation that could otherwise sabotage your health and your energy level. That's one reason why the Saint-Tropez Diet will keep you feeling constantly energized as you improve your looks and your health.

The Saint-Tropez Diet is not just about eating more omega-3 essential fatty acids. The other vital ingredient is retinol, or vitamin A. As we learned earlier, the PPARs are stimulated by the combination of omega-3 essential fatty acids and retinoic acid (which comes from vitamin A). The combination is the secret—and ensures that the omega-3s will be effective.

THE Saint Tropez Diet

Myths and Facts about Food and Dieting

Dieters have received many mixed messages about how to lose weight and stay healthy. Some of these messages, while well-intentioned, have no scientific basis in fact. Actually, some of them will interfere with your ability to lose weight and combine foods for their maximum health benefits. Here are a few myths.

> *Myth:* Whole milk is loaded with saturated fat and should be avoided by anyone who wants to lose weight.
> *Truth:* Consuming small amounts of whole milk or whole milk products offers important health benefits.

Milk is a wonderful and healthy food. It has a host of ingredients that actually support life. It contains all the vitamins we need to live except vitamin C and iron. Whole milk has gotten a bad rap because almost 70 percent of the fat in milk is saturated. Accordingly, skim and nonfat milk have become popular as less fattening sources of calcium.

Decades ago, skim milk was just a byproduct of the dairy industry. When milk fats were skimmed off of whole milk to create cream and butter, what was left over is what we call skim milk. At first the dairy industry had no idea how to sell this stuff, so they added sugar and cocoa to create chocolate milk, which was marketed for children. But not only does this just add sugar to children's diets, it turns out that children need milk fats for brain and body development.

We now know that it is the milk fats themselves that contain the vitamins in milk. In addition, the primary vitamins in milk, A and D, are fat-soluble, which means they must arrive encased in fat in order for the body to use them. In the 1970s and 1980s, the milk industry began to add vitamins A and D back into skim and nonfat milk, but without the fat, the body may not absorb these vitamins as effectively. In any case, whole milk is only about 4 percent fat, so a glass of milk gives you only 8 grams of saturated fat. If you had to give up all but 8 grams of saturated fat from your diet, I would recommend that those 8 grams come from whole milk.

Also, conjugated linoleic acid (CLA), one of the fatty acids that make up milk fat, helps the body shed fat. Although no one can tell if it is the only player, it is certainly one of the factors contributing to the recent studies showing that dairy consumption can lead to weight loss. CLA is found primarily in the fatty acids in organic whole milk, particularly in the milk of grass-fed cows.

As with any food, you don't want to overdo it, but if your milk intake is relatively small, such as a single glass per day, then whole milk and the vitamins it brings to your system is a healthy choice. This is true for all dairy products, especially yogurt, but be careful with cheese and cream, which are of course very high in fat.

> *Myth:* Bread, rice, and pasta are bad for you because they raise your blood sugar and make you fat.
>
> *Truth:* Whole grain foods, including multigrain bread, brown rice, and whole wheat pasta, have a host of health benefits.

Whole grains are an ancient source of nutrition, one that offers many important health benefits. A grain has three distinct parts. The germ is the innermost seed of the grain. The outer hull contains the bran and helps protect the grain from insects and diseases. These two parts of the grain contain much of its nutritive value, including the vitamins, minerals, and several types of antioxidants, including lignans, which are phytoestrogens. They also contain fiber, which is vital for cardiovascular and digestive health. The middle part is called the endosperm and contains the starch that would feed the seed should it be planted. All three of these parts need to be included in any product that claims to be a good or excellent source of whole grains. If you take a box of pasta or a loaf of bread off the shelf and look at the list of ingredients, the first word should be "whole." If the first word is "refined" or "enriched," then the product is probably not made from whole grain at all.

According to the Dietary Guidelines for Americans, updated and published every five years by the United States Department of Agriculture, we should be eating three servings of whole grains per day. Sadly, most Americans consume less than one serving of whole grains per day, despite the fact that so many convenience foods claim to be "whole wheat" or whole grain products.

If the whole grain is so nutritious, why was it ever refined? As with whole milk, the nutrients in whole grains fell victim to the needs of mass production. In order to make bread, rice, and pasta that could sit on supermarket shelves for weeks without growing mold, manufacturers removed the parts of the grain most likely to spoil, including the hull and much of the germ. In particular, they removed the outer edge of the wheat germ, called the bran, which was most prone to spoilage while the grain was stored. Unfortunately, the bran contains all of the fiber, vitamins, and minerals that make bread healthy and filling.

Not only do refined flours and grains not provide any nutrients, but they also have a negative effect on your insulin levels. Refined flour products tend to be low in fiber and high in starch, which means they have a high glycemic index. Foods with a high glycemic index spike your blood sugar and raise your insulin levels, which can increase your tendency to develop type 2 diabetes. And, since they are densely caloric foods with little filling fiber (which encourages you to eat more of it), refined flour products are a primary culprit in our obesity epidemic.

Thus, bread, rice, pasta, and other carbohydrates got a bad rap. Some diets tell you to give up all bread products. What they should be saying instead is to rethink the role that bread plays in your life. Every time you can forego a cookie or cheese cracker or some other densely caloric food based on refined white flour and turn instead to whole grains, you will be more likely to lose weight. In fact, several studies have shown that people who take in the highest amount of whole grains per day have a far easier time controlling their weight.

> **Myth:** Pouring fat-free salad dressing on your salad is a great way to cut calories and fat out of your diet.
> **Truth:** Eating vegetables served or cooked with olive oil, walnut oil, or canola oil can actually boost their nutritive value.

You know that you are supposed to eat your vegetables. That's the one stable piece of dietary advice that has not changed over the years.

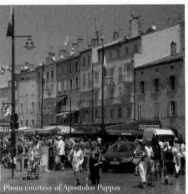

What has changed is our understanding of the role that oil plays in liberating the nutrients in those vegetables.

For example, the lycopene in tomatoes and tomato products is a powerful tool that fights cancer in general. And it's true that cooked tomato products, including jarred tomato sauce and salsas, retain all of the power of raw tomatoes to fight cancer. Studies are beginning to show that the lycopene in tomato products is better absorbed by the body when it is served with or cooked with oil. One study found that people who ate tomato products with oil had three times as much lycopene in their systems as people who consumed tomatoes that were steamed and puréed only, and served without oil.

Another study suggested that eating salads with fat-free dressing actually reduced the body's ability to make use of the healthy carotenoids (such as lycopene) when compared to salads with full-fat, oil-based dressings. A study conducted at Ohio State University concluded that adding avocado or avocado oil to salsa boosted the lycopene and carotenoid absorption by between two and four times the amount absorbed by those subjects eating avocado-free salsa.

This makes sense because lycopene, like all carotenoids, is fat-soluble, not water-soluble. That means that water can not liberate the nutrients in the food to make them bioavailable. Only oil can do that.

Even greens get a boost from cooking oil. Several recent studies have shown that absorption of the beta-carotene in green leafy vegetables was increased by two to five times the amount available to those who ate the greens cooked with no oil. Also, the subjects eating greens cooked in oil had a greater ability to absorb and produce vitamin A from those vegetables.

There's no need to assume that these vegetables must be drenched in oil in order to liberate their nutrients. In some studies, even small amounts of oil were effective in boosting carotenoid absorption. As long as some oil is present, the meal will become more nutritious. So feel free to enjoy full-fat salad dressings made with a combination of walnut oil and olive oil.

> **Myth:** Nuts are bad for dieters because they are so fattening.
> **Truth:** Actually, nuts have many important benefits, including their high omega-3 essential fatty acid content. When paired with their high levels of vitamin E, they become the perfect health food.

Vitamin E and omega-3s coexist in certain foods, such as nuts, seeds, and whole grains. Separately, they have many benefits, as discussed in earlier chapters. Together, they work to form a crucial antioxidant force that fights systemic inflammation and premature aging. In particular, vitamin E fights the oxidation of fat molecules traveling in the system. Consuming vitamin E, in the form of tocopherols, which are found in nuts and whole grains, can help protect the unsaturated fat circulating in your system and keep it from becoming oxidized or toxic to your system. Still, vitamin E needs the presence of omega-3 oils in order to become an antioxidant. Vitamins are cofactors in chemical reactions; that is, they facilitate specific reactions but can't cause the reactions to happen on their own. Consumed in tablet form, vitamin E is far less effective because it does not necessarily have omega-3s to act upon to deliver their antioxidative benefits. Rather than taking a vitamin E tablet, you would be better off eating a handful of nuts.

> **Myth:** Boiling vegetables destroys their nutrients.
> **Truth:** Cooking some vegetables does not harm them as much as we think.

According to raw food enthusiasts, vegetables need to be consumed in their natural form in order to be most nutritious. Actually, several studies refute this notion. An unpublished study at Rutgers University found that boiling cruciferous vegetables (such as broccoli) actually breaks down the cellulose and releases more of its minerals. After cooking, iron becomes more soluble and more easily absorbed by the body. While it's true that boiling broccoli and similar vegetables may reduce much of the vitamin C in the vegetable, this should not be a major concern. Vitamin C is certainly not the only reason to eat broccoli; in fact, it may be a minor player among the phytonutrients and other substances that make broccoli and similar vegetables such potent cancer-fighting foods.

And, as we've seen, the vitamins in some vegetables are better absorbed if they are cooked in oil.

Myth: Meat has no redeeming nutritional value. If you want to lose weight and be healthier, you should become a vegetarian.

Truth: Meat contains several important peptides, which are chains or groups of amino acids that form a complex nutritional substance. These exist only in meats and cannot be replicated in any other food. Proteins are polypeptide molecules (or consist of multiple polypeptide subunits).

Some people believe that mad cow disease was definitive proof that man should not be eating cows. The truth, of course, is much more complicated. Actually, the study of mad cow disease and how it is replicated has provided researchers with important information on how peptides from meat behave in our systems.

The epidemic developed in part because the cows were being fed a diet that contained some beef byproducts. In a sense, certain cows had become cannibals. Their brains became diseased because they consumed beef products made from animals that had that same disease.

This could never have happened if the beef peptides actually behaved in the cow's system the way scientists assumed that they did. Scientists have always assumed that meat peptides are broken down

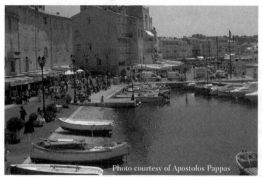

Photo courtesy of Apostolos Pappas

by the body into amino acids. Scientists assumed that all of the peptides were broken down into 20 amino acids, from which the body synthesizes new proteins. In fact, mad cow disease proves that certain peptides survive the digestive process and circulate through the system, eventually heading to the brain. There, the information in the peptides is taken up and utilized by the brain intact. Remember, too, that peptides are ligands, molecules that change the chemical formation of other molecules and alter their ability to function in other chemical reactions. Perhaps the peptides from meats offer important information to your cells and help regulate certain processes. If we consume vegetable proteins only, we may be missing out on these important peptides and their health benefits.

Even in the Provençal diet and the Mediterranean diet, meat is present. We should eat it in small amounts, rather than the huge steaks and burgers common in the Western diet. But a small amount of meat does have important nutritive value.

Myth: All oils rich in omega-6 essential fatty acids are bad for you.
Truth: Conjugated linoleic acid, found in whole dairy products and in modified safflower oil, is an important weight loss tool.

Conjugated linoleic acid (CLA) is a substance found naturally in animal meats and in cow's milk. Some recent studies have suggested that CLA has cancer-fighting properties and may be a powerful tool in weight management.

Researchers at Cornell boosted the CLA content of butter until it had 8 times the normal amount. When this butter was fed to rats with various forms of cancer, they showed improvement in that those rats given the CLA enhanced butter had significantly less tumor growth than those in the control group. These same researchers are testing CLA and its effects in fighting atherosclerosis.

Aside from whole milk dairy products, CLA is also readily available in products and supplements made from modified safflower oil. These seem to have some ability to help people maintain a healthier weight. In one study, healthy overweight adults were given one of these CLA supplements every day for 12 months. Those in the study group lost weight while maintaining their lean muscle mass. In some cases, participants reduced their weight by as much as 9 percent without altering their lifestyle in any other way.

The supplements may work by decreasing the amount of fat stored after eating, increasing the rate at which fat breaks down in the fat cells, increasing the rate of fat metabolism and decreasing the number of fat cells in the body—meaning that it works much like an omega-3 essential fatty acid.

Because CLA is available naturally in whole milk products and meat products, it is possible that taking in small amounts of these foods can give you many of the same effects. So many times, nutritionists have told people that whole milk and beef contain dangerous saturated fats, and they do. But they may also contain enough CLA to mitigate some of these effects.

Researchers from Ohio University have also reported that despite the fact that CLA is not an omega-3 essential fatty acid it activates the same fat-burning PPAR receptors that omega-3 activates. Probably that could be one of the reasons that this unusual fatty acid offers weight loss, fat-burning, and other anti-inflammatory benefits.

> **Myth:** Beef, pork, and chicken are all the same, regardless of their source. None of them is a great source of omega-3 essential fatty acids.
> **Truth:** Animals that have had a healthy and varied diet provide meat that is far more nutritious than animals fed only starchy grains.

There has been a revolution in the marketing of whole foods. Now consumers have access to free-range chickens and eggs from those chickens. These products are even being marketed as having more omega-3 essential fatty acids, and they do.

In nature, animals eat a widely varied diet of grasses and grains.

When meat became a mass-produced commodity, ranchers began to use the cheapest and most fattening grains to prepare animals for slaughter. As a result these animals consumed a very bland diet of hybrid corn, which is loaded with omega-6 essential fatty acids and virtually devoid of the healthier omega-3s, found in green leafy vegetables and plants. These animals are fattened up in part because they are starved for healthy fatty acids, and the deficit in their diet gets passed on to us whenever we eat these animals. Fish raised in farms has also been fed a controlled and artificial diet that will sharply reduce the omega-3 essential fatty acids it contains.

Animals like lamb and sheep that cannot be restrained to an artificial diet and must always graze on grass have a much higher content of omega-3s than pigs and cows, which are generally restricted to a diet of modified grains. Even feta and other cheeses based on sheep's or goat's milk have a high omega-3 content. The taste of wild game meats, such as venison and quail, may take some getting used to but will widen the variety of food in your diet.

By buying wild-caught seafood and grass-fed meats, you are increasing the healthy fatty acids in your diet and increasing your ability to lose weight.

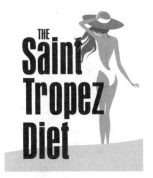

THE

Saint Tropez Diet

CHAPTER

7

Why Wine Is Good for Your Diet

The purpose of this chapter is not to suggest that drinking wine will help you to lose weight, but rather to inform you about the role that wine plays in the culture of Saint-Tropez and potentially in your kitchen. In Provence and throughout the Mediterranean, people easily maintain a healthy weight while consuming a glass or two of wine nearly every day. In fact, many of the people who live in France would consider a life without wine to be an unacceptable deprivation. In France, wine is ingrained in the culture as a healthy and natural substance, the consumption of which is a pleasurable, creative experience. That overall sense that food and wine in moderation combine to make a meal a celebratory experience is a key component to staying healthy and thin. Here's why.

The Culture of Wine

In America, many people often refer to wine simply as an alcoholic drink, a type of drug. In France and throughout the Mediterranean, a bottle of wine is considered to be a living substance that is constantly changing and maturing inside the bottle until the moment it is opened. Once wine has been poured into a glass, it begins to oxidize, much like the flesh of an apple that has been cut open reacts to oxygen in the air by turning brown. In the case of wine, it is said to "open up," meaning that the flavors briefly mature and become more vibrant. In this way, each sip can taste slightly different than any other.

If you have studied a particular wine before you drink it, if you know about the soil and climate in which the grapes were grown, if

59

you know the philosophies of the winemaker toward his craft, then you can anticipate some of its tastes and effects before you take the first sip. This moment of knowledge and anticipation is about as far from consuming a drug as you can get. If you can bring this type of anticipation and knowledge to the food you eat, then it will become more difficult to treat food like a drug, too.

In France, and particularly in Provence, people bring the same passion and understanding to the food they eat. If each bite is a sacred experience to be enjoyed alongside good wine and good conversation, then food is something that can fully satisfy, even in smaller portions. That is how a change in attitude toward food and wine can help you maintain a healthy weight.

Wine in Provence

Provence is like any other region of France in that it has its own distinctive range of wine varieties. In this case, the varieties are influenced by the Mediterranean climate of the area, which offers ample sunshine, far more than a vine could ever need to produce grapes. The extreme south of France also has fairly mild, dry winters. The northern wind, known as the mistral, abuses the vines in Provence, but also helps protect them against some diseases common to vineyards. In this way, it is easier for some winemakers to produce organic wines.

Much of the wine produced in Provence is rosé, meaning that the red grape skins are allowed to soak, or macerate, with the juice for a few hours until they have given the juice a slightly pink color. Then the skins are removed and the winemaking continues without them. These pale, dry wines pair well with the olive oil and garlic common in Provençal fare. Still, some wine snobs dislike the rosés of Provence, saying that they only taste good when well-chilled and sipped on a searing beach. The red wines of Provence, including those from such areas, or appellations, as Bandol, Bellet, and Cassis have a fine reputation as spicy and interesting wines that pair perfectly with the cuisine of the region. Still, winemakers in Provence produce wines of many varieties.

If you're new to wines, the wines of Provence are a wonderful place to begin your education. But don't limit yourself to them, by any means. Since the Saint-Tropez Diet emphasizes flavors from the whole Mediterranean region, why not try some Greek, southern Italian, Spanish, or Portuguese wines, too? Wines from other regions of France (Bordeaux, Bourgogne, Loire, Alsace) and European countries like Germany and Austria also match wonderfully with this type of cuisine. And once you've gotten a sense of the types of wine you like, try varietals from Australia, North America, South America, South Africa, or any other vineyards you think you might enjoy. Part of the fun of learning about wines is in learning the differences between wines from different countries and different regions. The important thing is to savor the flavors and enjoy.

Many diets don't allow alcohol of any kind, because alcoholic drinks can be more densely packed with calories than other kinds of

CHOOSING WINE FOR DINNER

People always say that wine should complement food, but without having studied wine for a lifetime, that may seem difficult to do. The best strategy is to think of wine as a side dish to your meal. It brings a group of flavors that can act in harmony with what you're eating. Remember, too, that you probably know more than you think about which flavors will taste good together. After all, if you were preparing a pasta dish with a heavy cream sauce, you probably wouldn't choose to drink lemonade with it. The extreme tartness of the lemons would make the cream sauce taste funny. So you should choose a wine that has flavors that complement the flavors in your meal.

A second consideration is to balance the weight of the wine with the weight of the food you serve. If you are serving a hearty meat stew, then a light white wine, such as a Sauvignon Blanc, will be overpowered by the food. By contrast, a lightly-flavored fish dish would be drowned by the hearty flavors of a Cabernet Sauvignon or a Syrah.

foods. After all, the primary goal of many diets is to cut calories. According to this reasoning, perhaps skipping the wine is best. But in Saint-Tropez, as in many French and Mediterranean cultures, wine is often called "the water of life." To deny oneself a glass of wine at dinner in order to lose weight is too much to ask. Accordingly, the Saint-Tropez Diet makes an allowance for a glass of wine at dinner in at least some of its phases.

If you want to add elegant notes in a celebratory moment during your diet, try Extra Brut Chamagne. Extra Brut, Brut Sauvage, Ultra Brut, Brut Integral or Brut Zero are types of champagne in which little or no sugar is added; they have less than 0.6% of residual sugar per liter. This champagne will be very dry (the less sugar a wine—especially a white wine-has, the more dry it is) and have a lower glycemic index than most wines.

It's true, of course, that wine must be enjoyed in moderation. And in moderation, wine offers many well-documented health benefits.

Photo courtesy of Apostolos Pappas

Health Benefits of Wine

Numerous studies have outlined the health benefits of moderate alcohol consumption. In the Physician's Health Study, which tracked the health of 22,000 doctors over the age of 40 for 11 years, found a 30 to 35 percent reduction in heart attack and angina in moderate drinkers over nondrinkers. A much larger study conducted by the American Cancer Society followed the health of more than 489,000 men and women over the age of 30 and found that over 9 years there was a 30 to 40 percent reduced risk of heart disease-related death in those same moderate drinkers compared to nondrinkers. In these two studies, researchers did not differentiate between wine or beer consumption, which may indicate that some health benefits can be realized from the alcohol itself.

Still, wine seems to be unique in that it contains several components that may have health benefits. Because wine is made from grapes, it contains many of the same antioxidants found in grapes, particularly in the grape skins. Red wine may contain even more of these antioxidants and phytochemicals than white wine because the fermentation process is carried out in part with the nutrient-rich grape skins intact.

These antioxidants and phytochemicals help prevent heart attacks by:

- Reducing the rate at which LDL cholesterol (bad cholesterol) becomes oxidized, and therefore harmful, to the arteries.
- Increasing the level of HDL cholesterol particles (good cholesterol) in the system.
- Relaxing the arteries so that they are less likely to constrict and pinch off blood flow to the heart muscle.
- Moderating the blood clotting response that can be overactive in people with heart disease.

In addition to powerful antioxidants, wine also contains polyphenols, which help stimulate the body's immune system and antibacterial responses. These effects can help battle certain forms of cancer.

What's In Wine?

THE CLASSIC APERITIF

In Saint-Tropez, as in the rest of Provence, you will be invited to drink a certain classic aperitif to get you in the mood for lunch or dinner. This anise-flavored drink, called pastis, is amber colored until it is mixed with water, when it turns white. That is why it is sometimes called "The Milk of Provence." Some cafés serve their pastis straight, with no water. Some mix it with grenadine and call it a tomato. Others add mint syrup and call it a parrot. Whatever its name, the anise liqueur boasts a knee-buckling 45 percent alcohol, so it is best to try just one. You can find pastis in most wine and spirits stores. Look for Pernod-Ricard, Pastis, or Ouzo (the Greek version).

Wine contains a group of substances called flavonoids, a type of polyphenol, which are water-soluble plant pigments, the chemicals that help give vegetables their color. These flavonoids are particularly concentrated in the skins of grapes. Those

CHEF MARIE-ANNICK'S STORY

I was exposed to wine at a very early age. In France, it is not unusual to see a bottle of wine at the dinner table. When I was 10 years old, my parents decided to introduce me to wine by adding a drop to my full glass of water. We were at my grandparents' house for a family reunion. That single drop of wine made me suddenly realize that I was no longer considered a kid and that I was old enough to start to experience new pleasures of life. I was told that the older I got, the less water would be mixed with the wine.

With the experience came the speech, in which I was told to appreciate, respect, and treasure wine. I was told to deguster *or savor the wine, and not to gobble it up. I was told that savoring wine brings many joys, but abusing it will cause serious consequences to my health.*

My parents told me what is reasonable to drink, a glass or two at the most, in the same way that they had told me what is reasonable to eat. In France, parents serve their children food until they are 10 years old. After that, children serve

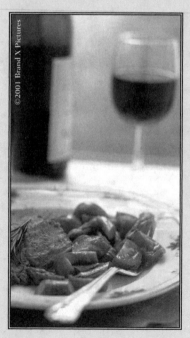

themselves. My brother, similarly, was given the right to pour wine into glasses when he was 14. My parents gave me examples of tragedies that come from alcohol abuse, such as car accidents, divorce, loss of job. I was told to practice self-discipline and to look out for others who drink too much.

I was taught the culture and the rituals of buying and serving wine. In France, the man in every household opens and serves the wine, but the woman must know how to purchase wine. Both must know how to pair foods with wine. I was also told that learning about wine would take me many years and involve all of my senses. If I was prudent and diligent, the adventure could last a lifetime.

As a family, we made many trips to wineries. During these trips, I learned about grape growing, winemaking, and how to respect the work of the winemakers. I learned to look at a bottle, its art and information. I learned to see, smell, and taste wine. I saw how to store wine at the wineries, but also at my father's cave. Finally, I was taught how to serve wine. Through these trips and rituals, I came to understand that there is nothing better than sharing wine with others and that a pairing of great food and wine tops the list of the best pleasures in life.

While shopping, my parents would educate me on how the bottles are stored, which wine to select and why. Sometimes my mom would figure out at the store what she would cook for dinner, and then we would go choose a wine. Other times, she would tell me she felt like drinking a certain wine, and then we would select food accordingly.

The education of my senses was also done at the table with many different wines and food. My grandparents, aunts and uncles, along with my parents' friends, all contributed to that education. We had games of who could guess aromas and what food would go well with it by just smelling the wine. Needless to say, it was lots of fun, and I didn't miss any occasion I was given to learn more. Through all these experiences came excitement, but also the realization of so many new pleasures.

I realized the importance of such an education, with its loving guidelines and beautiful memories, as I grew older, when I moved away from home and started to entertain or go out to restaurants. This education is part of our social environment in France. I also thought at that time that if I ever had children, I would want the same for my kids. Isn't it how the traditions are passed?

skins also create the tannins in red wine, which is where the flavonoids are found in abundance.

Scientists have identified thousands of flavonoids. Of these, three are known to be in red wine:

Resveratrol. This is a chemical that protects grapes and some other plants against fungal infections. Scientists proved that it also acts as an antioxidant and may be an anticoagulant. It may have anti-cancer properties as well. Resveratrol is also found in raspberries and peanuts.

Quercetin. This substance is found in many foods, including apples (particularly their skins), tea, and several kinds of berries. Consuming a lot of vegetables rich in quercetin has been linked with improved overall health, decreased rates of heart disease and cancer, and even reduced rates of lung disease.

Catechins. These are found in relatively high quantities in green and black tea and in somewhat smaller quantities in red wine. They are powerful antioxidants that protect against free radicals in the body. White wine has not been studied to the same extent as red wine, but may also contain some benefits.

Options for Nondrinkers

Not everyone drinks alcohol. Certainly not everyone needs to drink alcohol in order to realize the health benefits of these nutraceuticals in wine. Nondrinkers can eat grapes or drink grape juice and will get most, or perhaps all, of the benefits of these chemicals. These nutraceuticals are also found in many of the so-called superfoods, including blueberries, broccoli, tea, chocolate, and members of the onion family.

If you currently avoid alcohol for whatever reason, there is no need to start drinking wine in order to follow this diet or to attain the health benefits described in this chapter. If you do enjoy a glass of wine occasionally, you will be taking in these benefits automatically.

Many of the substances identified here as beneficial, including resveratrol and quercetin, are available in supplement form. Be warned, however, that supplements are not regulated for their contents by the FDA. Also, there are no current studies available to inform consumers of the safe levels of these supplements. Scientists are also learning that the absorption of these chemicals depends heavily on their source. They may need to be ingested in whole food form in order to work at all. These chemicals could be toxic in high doses, or they could do nothing. As always, it is better to consume whole foods than to turn to isolated chemicals and flavonoids in supplement form.

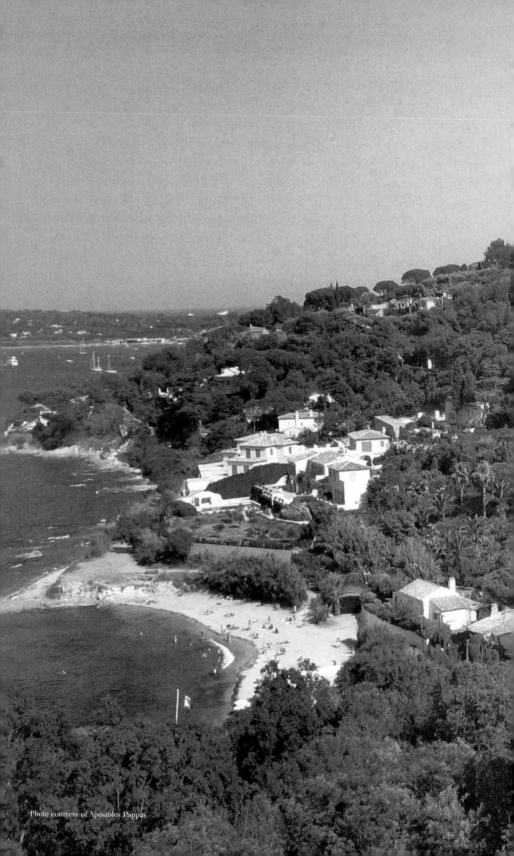

Meal Plans for the Saint-Tropez Diet

Now that you have a good understanding of why the Saint-Tropez Diet will help you lose weight, fight disease, and boost your energy with a delicious mix of fresh and wholesome foods, it's time to put these principles into action.

This section presents an eight-week meal plan to get you started on the path to a lifetime of savoring gourmet meals and good health. Packed with foods rich in omega-3 essential fatty acids and brimming with vitamin A and other vital nutraceuticals, this plan is designed so that you never feel as if you're on a diet. And don't worry! Although it may seem like a lot of work at first, you'll soon be rewarded by the discovery of a whole new world of spices and flavors.

There are lots of ways you can customize the diet according to your weight loss goals, cooking ability, personal tastes, time commitments, and exercise levels. Be sure to review the four basic principles of the diet, and feel free to mix and match recipes according to these principles.

begin

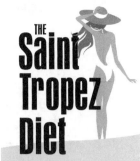

How to Use the
Saint-Tropez Meal Plans

Now that you understand why the Saint-Tropez Diet works to help you lose weight, it's time to put the diet into practice! In fact, even if you don't understand why it works, you can still make the diet work for you. In order to reach the optimal ratio of omega-6 to omega-3 essential fatty acids (about 4 to 1) and thus turbocharge your cells fat-burning receptors, all you need to do is to follow these four simple principles:

1. **Eat more foods that contain relatively large amounts of healthy unsaturated fats, especially omega-3 essential fatty acids.** These include wild salmon, sardines, herring, anchovies, and other oily fish; walnuts, flaxseeds (crushed to release the oil); and oils such as olive oil, canola oil, walnut oil, and flaxseed oil. In this diet, you will have one to two servings of these foods per day. Be careful not to overdo your nut and oil consumption though, since they can add calories quickly.

2. **Eat foods rich in vitamin A together with foods containing omega-3 essential fatty acids when possible.** Vitamin A is found in carrots, squash, beets, sweet potatoes, spinach, red and yellow bell peppers, pumpkin, tomatoes, cantaloupes, mangoes, apricots, and other red, orange, and yellow vegetables and fruit. A serving of two per day ensures the daily recommended allowance of your vitamin A needs.

3. **Eliminate foods in which the omega-6 to omega-3 essential fatty acids ratio is unhealthy or in which there are no healthy unsaturated fats at all.** These include all convenience foods, all foods from vending machines, and all baked goods made with refined white flour and sugar, and red

meat. Instead, opt for whole grains (three to four servings a day) and lean meats such as free-range chicken, turkey, duck, lamb, and grass-fed beef. Because these meats tend to be higher in saturated fats include three or fewer servings per week.

4. **Eat plenty of fruits and vegetables that are rich in nutraceuticals with antioxidant activity in order to counteract the oxidative effect of fats.** Ideally, you will be eating fresh fuits and vegetables, especially dark green leafy vegetables like spinach and collard greens, every day. You should aim for six to eight servings of fruits and vegetables.

The following chapters contain some suggested menus to help you ease into this new way of eating. The menus are organized into the following phases.

Phase 1: Introducing Good Fats and Fresh Ingredients (Week 1)—approximately 1,600 calories per day. This phase focuses on replacing as many of the saturated fats in your diet with omega-3 essential fatty acids found in canola, olive, and walnut oil, salmon and other oily fish, and flaxmeal and other nuts and seeds.

Phase 2: Balancing Diet and Lifestyle (Week 2)—approximately 1,450 calories per day. In this phase, you will continue to add foods rich in omega-3s to your diet but reduce your overall calorie intake slightly. If you don't already exercise, you will want to start walking or other mild exercise several times a week. If you do already exercise, increase your frequency or intensity slightly.

Phase 3: Reaching Your Ideal Weight (Weeks 3 to 6)—approximately 1,300 to 1,400 calories per day. This is the core of the weight loss program, in which you simultaneously reduce your calorie intake and exercise more intensely in order to burn more calories. However, as you'll see, it is easiest to lose weight if you do not feel deprived. So you may find it necessary to eat more because you are exercising more.

Phase 4: Maintaining a Healthy Lifestyle (Weeks 7 to 8)— approximately 1,500 to 1,600 calories per day. In the last two weeks of the program, you'll continue to increase your daily intake of omega-3s and vitamin A to optimize your fat-burning receptors. This phase

A NOTE ABOUT SNACKS

In recent years, some experts have been touting the importance of eating meals throughout the day in order to prevent fluctuations in blood sugar and energy levels and to keep your metabolism humming. While there may be some truth to this, there is certainly no need to stick to a strict timeline to eat every three hours or four hours or whatever. In other words, if you don't need to snack, you don't have to. What is important is that you try to consume most of your calories earlier in the day, when you are most active, rather than skipping or skimping on breakfast and lunch and then gorging at dinner.

You'll see that we've included a snack between lunch and dinner every day in the meal plan. If having a midafternoon snack keeps you from feeling deprived and keeps your energy levels high, then by all means, have the snack as indicated in the meal plan. But if instead you tend to get hungrier in the morning, have the snack before lunch. Or if you find that the lunches we've indicated don't fill you up, have the snack as part of your lunch. And again, if you're feeling deprived, have an additional snack. Just make sure your snack is full of healthy omega-3s and nutraceuticals, rather than omega-6s, and try to avoid snacking after dinner.

should be at a calorie level you can maintain for the rest of your life to stay at a healthy weight, boost your metabolism, reduce your chance of disease, and still enjoy your food. Keep in mind that, while you want to practice portion control, you don't want to feel deprived, so again, feel free to add calories to suit your circumstances within the principles stated above. In this phase, you can cut back on your exercise frequency or intensity slightly, but you never want to stop moving.

As you can see, this meal plan is based on a 1,300-calorie menu at its strictest point. The number of calories you need to function varies according to your gender, age, height, metabolic rate, and many other factors. And of course, the number of calories you need to lose weight also varies; in addition to the factors mentioned above, it also depends on

A NOTE ABOUT EXERCISE

As we noted, if you lived in Saint-Tropez, you would walk a lot more than you probably do now. You would also probably enjoy gardening, regularly tote heavy bags of groceries home from the market, and take a stroll after dinner. You might also go swimming or dancing or play badminton and la boule. In other words, you would naturally be getting mild exercise all day long.

But if you aren't already regularly active, it can help to start a regular exercise routine. Walking, as we've noted, is a great way to start if you haven't exercised before. But eventually you'll want to incorporate several different types of exercise into your routine, including:

- Aerobic (or endurance) exercises, which increase your breathing and heart rate. This helps you maintain a healthy weight, improves your stamina for everyday tasks, and keeps your heart and lungs healthy. Aim for 3 to 5 days of aerobic exercise, with about 30 minutes of exercise on each day. Warm up before starting your activity, and cool down afterward for 5 to 10 minutes.

- Strength training exercises, which build muscle. This helps you burn more calories, firms and shapes your body, boosts your metabolism, and increases bone density. Aim for 2 to 6 days of strength training exercise, for 20 to 60 minutes each time. Warm up with 5 to 10 minutes of light aerobic activity, and avoid working the same muscle groups 2 days in a row.

- Flexibility exercises, which stretch your muscles and surrounding tissues. This helps prevent injuries and maintains your range of motion as you get older. You should stretch after you do either aerobic or strength training exercise, or any time you feel you need it. Some studies have shown stretching before exercise to be ineffective or even harmful, but these studies are not conclusive. Pay attention to your body, and don't overdo your stretches.

- Balance exercises, which improve your balance and coordination. This also helps prevent injuries and falls. You can

> *incorporate balance challenges into your strength training exercises by doing exercises on different surfaces or on one leg.*
>
> *Whatever you do, though, don't overdo it! While mild exercise has immense health benefits, excessive or strenuous exercise can lead to injuries and stress. It's best to check with your doctor, work with a trainer, or at least consult a fitness book written by reputable professionals before you start your exercise program.*

your activity level and how much weight you want to lose. (Men especially tend to require a higher calorie count.) We've chosen the 1,300-calorie menu as a base because that's the lowest level we'd recommend for most adults; any lower, and you're likely to miss out on key nutrients.

But, as we've been emphasizing all along, the point of this diet is not to count calories. It is easiest to lose weight and keep it off if you never feel deprived. So if you find that you're hungry during any of the phases of the meal plan, simply add a healthy snack or two to add 100 to 200 calories. Remember that when you consume more omega-3s along with more natural nutraceuticals, especially vitamin A, you will be sending messages to your body to burn fat even at these higher calorie counts. However, when you consume the wrong type of fat, it will have the opposite effect and your body will store fat instead.

Similarly, if you find that you need more than one or two weeks to get used to eating more fresh foods or cooking more often or exercising on a more regular basis, then by all means, feel free to extend Phases 1 and 2. Again, you will still be burning fat in those phases. Also, studies show that people who lose weight gradually are more likely to keep it off, so it may be better in the long run to stretch out the first two phases a bit.

New Foods and New Cooking

When you try any new diet, you will find that the greatest challenge is in learning to shop for and prepare new foods. In this diet, the entrees, snacks, and salads sometimes call for numerous unfamiliar (but very healthy) foods. You will want to scan the recipes and shop for several days in advance. However, since we are emphasizing fresh ingredients, you'll probably find that you can't shop too far in advance, since many of the fish, vegetables, and fruits stay fresh only for a few days. This will take some getting used to, but since you'll also be buying less with each trip, you should find that it doesn't really take much more time or cost much more than shopping for a week or two at a time. If you really need to shop for a week or so in advance, though, opt for frozen fruits, vegetables, and fish; they tend to have fewer additives than canned or shelf-stable foods.

You may also want to prepare and freeze a couple of soups (don't freeze cream-based soups, though) or other recipes (even many of the fish dishes) on a day when you have more time in order to save time during those days when you are busy. Most recipes include information on how to store and freeze leftovers. Although, again, it's healthier and tastier to cook with fresh ingredients for each meal, we know that's not always possible in our busy society. When you're in a rush, homemade leftovers are a better option than fast food or canned or prepackaged meals.

Remember also that you can modify the recipes if you can't find a certain type of fish or a specific vegetable. Again, most recipes indicate alternate ingredients. But you should also feel free to experiment. If you visit your local farmers market and see a green leafy vegetable that's unfamiliar to you, for instance, try that instead of spinach in your Spinach with Pine Nuts and Raisins. One tip: Some vegetables are wonderful raw but many, such as zucchini and cauliflower, may be a little hard to swallow. If you don't like a vegetable raw, try steaming it lightly and drizzling a little olive oil or lemon juice on it. The cooking process breaks down the starches in these vegetables into sugars, which are a little tastier. Then you can snack on it or add it to salads, as you would a raw vegetable. As long as you stick to fresh ingredients, you will continue to reap the health benefits of the diet, and you will learn to appreciate and enjoy your food the French way.

Similarly, you'll see that not all of the recipes in this book are included in the meal plan. The sample menus here are just that—samples—so feel free to mix and match with other recipes to suit your tastes and your lifestyle. See the table below for some ideas on how to do that.

#1: EAT MORE OMEGA-3S			
FOODS			
Tuna	Wild Salmon	Sardines	Herring
Anchovies	Walnuts	Flaxseeds (crushed to release the oil)	Olive Oil
Canola Oil	Walnut Oil	Flaxseed Oil	

RECIPES

Rye Bread with Cream Cheese and Salmon

Salmon and Asparagus Omelet

Pasta with Anchovies

Broiled Salmon with Dill

Tuna with Balsamic Vinegar

Trout Greek Style

Trout with Almonds

Sablefish with Honey and Thyme

*Swordfish with Capers

*Hake with Leek Fondue

*Sardines and Spinach au Gratin

Stuffed Herrings with Potatoes and Onions

*Monkfish Provence Style

*Sea Bass with Ginger and Lime

*Mackerels with Garlic Cloves

*Mackerels with Mushrooms

*Cod Fish with Ratatouille and Feta Cheese

Salmon and Fennel Papilotte

*Salmon with Orange Sauce

*Salmon with Basil Aioli

*Dogfish with Spicy Red Wine Sauce

*Tuna Basque Style

*Baked Sardines with Greens

Tuna Daube

Sea Bream with Saffron

*Ocean Perch with Bell Pepper Coulis

Red Snapper with Basil and Oregano

Sardines Escabèche Style

Fish Soup

Smoked Duck Salad with Raspberry Vinaigrette

*Artichokes and Fava Beans Salad

*Leeks with Walnut Vinaigrette

*Tomato and Basil Salad

*Carrot Salad with Lemon

*Chicken Salad with Celery and Apple

*Fisherman Salad

*Niçoise Salad

*Mesclun Greens with Goat Cheese

*Curly Endive Greek Style

*Lentil Salad

*Baby Bell Peppers with Tuna

Olive Paste and Red Bell Pepper Bruschetta

Pesto and Salmon Bruschetta

Apple and Walnut Bruschetta

Stuffed Mushrooms with Tapenade

Cherry Tomatoes with Cod Fish

Monkfish with Nut Chutney

Smoked Salmon Rolls

*Grilled Vegetables with Anchovy Vinaigrette

*Broccoli with Pistachio Vinaigrette

Tuna Carpaccio with Pistachios

Eggplant Caviar

*Poached Red Mullet with Basil Sauce

*Sea Bream with Almonds and Edible Flowers

Sole Fillets with White Beans Velouté

*Thin Tart with Prime Tender Vegetables

* THESE RECIPES SERVE DOUBLE-DUTY WITH INGREDIENTS THAT CONTRIBUTE TO MORE THAN ONE PRINCIPLE.

NOTE : RECIPIES ARE LISTED IN ORDER OF THEIR APPEARANCE IN THE BOOK. SEE THE LIST OF RECIPES ON PAGE 313 FOR PAGE NUMBERS.

#2: EAT MORE VITAMIN A.

FOODS

Carrots	Squash	Beets	Sweet Potatoes
Spinach	Red and Yellow Bell Peppers	Pumpkin	Tomatoes

RECIPES

Omelet Provence Style

* Trout with Almonds

* Swordfish with Walnuts

* Hake with Leek Fondue

* Sardines and Spinach au Gratin

* Monkfish Provence Style

* Sea Bass with Ginger and Lime

* Mackerels with Garlic Cloves

* Mackerels with Mushrooms

* Cod Fish with Ratatouille and Feta Cheese

* Salmon with Orange Sauce

* Salmon with Basil Aioli

* Dogfish with Spicy Red Wine Sauce

* Tuna Basque Style

* Baked Sardines with Greens

* Ocean Perch with Bell Pepper Coulis

Beef Stew Provence Style

Pork Loin with Tomato Coulis

Chicken Breast with Garlic Cloves

Pork Roast with Figs

Cornish Hen with Olives

Gazpacho

Chickpea, Tomato, and Rice Soup

*Pumpkin Soup

Mushroom and Hazelnut Soup

Soup with Pistou

Carrot and Orange Soup

Melon with Figs and Prosciutto

* Artichokes and Fava Beans Salad

* Tomato and Basil Salad

* Carrot Salad with Lemon

* Fisherman Salad

* Niçoise Salad

* Mesclun Greens with Goat Cheese

* Curly Endive Greek Style

Squid and Roasted Bell Peppers Salad

* Baby Bell Peppers with Tuna

Tomato and Walnut Bruschetta

Cherry Tomatoes with Cod Fish

Smoked Salmon Rolls

*Spinach Boreks

Orange-Glazed Carrots

Spinach with Pine Nuts and Raisins

*Green Beans with Tomatoes

*Steamed Vegetables

* Grilled Vegetables with Anchovy Vinaigrette

*Swiss Chard Tagine

*Tomatoes Provence Style

*Vegetables Gratin with Thyme

*Stuffed Bell Peppers

Stuffed Eggplant

* Broccoli with Pistachio Vinaigrette

*Marinated Vegetables with Lemon Ratatouille

Tomatoes Napoleon

* Eggplant au Gratin

* Poached Red Mullet with Basil Sauce

* Thin Tart with Prime Tender Vegetables

* Sea Bream with Almonds

and Edible Flowers

FOODS

#3: EAT FEWER OMEGA 6S.

Whole grain, rather than refined

No convenience foods or foods from vending machines

No baked goods made with refined white flour and sugar

Lean and grass-fed meat rather than red meat

RECIPES

Whole Grain Bread with Laughing Cow Cheese, Pear, and Walnut

Whole Grain Bread with Almond Butter, Apricot Preserves, and Almond

Granola with Banana, Apple, and Walnut

Oatmeal with Almond, Apricot, Apple, and Mango

Muesli with Dried Fruit and Nuts

Wheat Bran Flakes with Berries and Raisins

Oat Bran Flax Muffin

Buckwheat Crêpes with Cottage Cheese, Berries, and Kiwi

Lamb Chops with Herbs

*Chicken Breast with Wild Mushrooms

Chicken Breast with Garlic Cloves

Stuffed Turkey Breast

Italian Style Cornish Hen with Olives

Lentil Soup

Lentil Salad

Risotto with Olives

The Apostolos Crêpes

Marie's Oatmeal Cookies

FOODS

#4: EAT MORE NUTRACEUTICALS

Fruits and vegetables

RECIPES

* Swordfish with Capers

* Sea Bream with Saffron

Duck Breast with Berries

*Chicken Breast with Wild Mushrooms

Pork Roast with Figs

Roasted Goose with Chestnuts

Rabbit Stew Greek Style

*Pumpkin Soup

*Carrot and Orange Soup

Beat and Fennel Soup

Onion Soup

Smoked Duck Salad with Raspberry Vinaigrette

*Carrot Salad with Lemon

* Chicken Salad with Celery and Apple

Beets with Walnuts

Stuffed Mushrooms with Tapenade

Porcini Mushrooms Provence Style

Couscous with Vegetables

* Spinach with Pine Nuts and Raisins

* Green Beans with Tomatoes

* Steamed Vegetables

*Grilled Vegetables with Anchovy Vinaigrette

* Swiss Chard Tagine

* Tomatoes Provence Style

* Vegetables Gratin with Thyme

*Stuffed Bell Peppers

*Broccoli with Pistachio Vinaigrette

*Marinated Vegetables with Lemon

Pasta with Sun-Dried Tomatoes and Artichoke

Potato Parsnip Purée

White Bean Stew

Wild Rice with Vegetables

Fruit Salad with Mint

Melon Soup

Stuffed Peaches

Figs Compote with Yogurt

Strawberries with Spicy Red Wine

The Aposotolos Crêpes with Strawberry Filling or Apple Filling

Poached Pears with Black Muscat

Baked Apples with Toasted Walnuts

Orange Salad with Champagne

*Eggplant Caviar

Nectarine with Raspberries and Fresh Verbena

You'll note that some recipes aren't categorized according to the four principles, but each recipe is nutritious and delicious, particularly when paired with a side dish with nutraceuticals or vitamin A-rich foods.

Here are some other ideas to vary the meal plans.

- Fresh fruit is the simplest, quickest, and healthiest snack or dessert.
- Most of the snacks all have about 100 calories. If you feel too hungry or deprived, have two or three snacks to add 200 to 300 calories.
- Have one serving of any of the following recipes as a side dish with lunch or dinner or as a snack to add about 200 calories: Gazpacho, Lentil Soup, Carrot and Orange Soup, Pumpkin Soup, Onion Soup, Trout Greek Style, Couscous with Vegetables, Spinach with Pine Nuts and Raisins, Marinated Vegetables with Lemon, Lentil Salad, or Basil and Tomato Salad.
- Have two servings of any of the following recipes to add 200 calories: Monkfish with Nut Chutney, Beet and Fennel Soup, Green Beans with Tomatoes, or Grilled Vegetables with Anchovy Vinaigrette.
- Add the following for 200 calories of healthy ingredients to your day: 1/4 cup of nuts; 1 cup of beans (kidney, black, chickpeas, lentils); 1 tablespoon of flax seed oil, walnut oil, or olive oil plus 2 servings of fruit; 2 tablespoons of nuts plus 2 servings of fruit (1 serving of fruit = 1 cup cut fruit, 1 cup berries, 1/2 cup canned fruit packed in juice or water, or 1 medium whole piece of fruit).

Forbidden and Not Quite Forbidden Foods

Although you shouldn't deprive yourself, there are some foods you should avoid entirely. Traditional fast foods are completely forbidden on this diet, as you might have guessed. Also forbidden are many of the so-called health foods and prepackaged convenience foods. Most people have a pantry of these items, and they will sabotage your efforts to lose weight and eat a healthier diet. These include:

- Anything you can buy in a vending machine (unless you are lucky enough to find a machine that dispenses yogurt or fruit)
- Highly processed foods

TIPS ON SELECTING FISH

Try to shop for fresh fish the day that you'll be serving it to ensure the best quality. Here are some guidelines for choosing the freshest catch.

- *Fish should have a shiny luster and a moist surface.*
- *The flesh should be sturdy with a little cushion that springs back when pressed.*
- *Scales should be clear and bright and intact, attached to the fish. Fresh fish sometimes have slightly red or pinkish scales.*
- *Avoid fish with sunken eyes; the eyes should appear bright.*
- *The odor should be fresh and mild.*
- *If you are buying steaks or fillets, look for a natural color, mild odor, and firm texture. Be wary of a shiny surface or thick moisture, which is usually a sign of spoilage.*
- *Avoid flavored fillets or steaks. The store usually uses this method to get rid of older, less fresh fish.*

Certain types of fish may contain higher levels of mercury (excess consumption of mercury can harm the brain, heart, kidney, and lungs). Don't let the fears of mercury contamination keep you from consuming seafood altogether, but rather choose fish known to have lower mercury levels and enjoy! It may be difficult to tell which fish have high levels of mercury because it often depends upon whether they came from polluted areas. But in general, these fish tend to have high mercury levels: king mackerel, shark, swordfish, and tilefish (golden bass or golden snapper).

These fish tend to have low mercury levels: anchovies, butterfish, catfish, clams, cod, crawfish, croaker (Atlantic), flatfish, haddock, hake, herring, jacksmelt, lobster (spiny), mackerel (North Atlantic), mackerel chub (Pacific), mullet, oysters, perch ocean, pickerel, Pollock, salmon (canned, fresh, frozen), sardine, scallops, shad (American), shrimp, squid, tilapia, trout (freshwater), tuna (canned, light), whitefish, and whiting.

- Sodas
- Frozen or microwave-ready-to-heat meals and snacks (except, of course, the ones you make yourself from our recipes)
- Anything containing high fructose corn syrup (read the labels and discard anything with this in it)
- Diet foods, particularly fat-free or low-fat desserts
- Sweetened cereals or "whole wheat breads" with a fiber content less than 3 grams per serving
- Fried foods
- Shelf-stable snacks (boxes of cheese crackers, bags of tortilla chips, and sports bars, even if they claim to be "all natural" or "organic") — the only shelf-stable snacks you should have are unsweetened dried fruits and unsalted nuts
- Fatty cuts of meat and deli meats
- Fat-free milk or yogurt

In addition, there are some foods that aren't completely forbidden—which, in fact, may be rich in nutrients that are good for you—but should be consumed only in moderation. The foods on this list shouldn't be eaten at every meal every day, but they can be enjoyed as treats. They include:

- Fruit juices (preferably 100 percent juice with no added sugar) — up to one cup per day (note that some are high in fiber and others rich in antioxidant activity)
- Full-fat cheese — one to two ounces per day
- Eggs — one per day, up to five per week
- Full-fat milk or yogurt — one to four times per week
- Wine — one to five times per week
- Chocolate (preferably dark) — one to four times per week

Because many of these foods are high in calories, be careful not to gorge on these. Also, many of these foods—especially fruit juices—may have added sugar, colorants, or preservatives. Read the labels carefully and stick, as much as possible, to whole foods.

You'll see, by the way, that in keeping with the Saint-Tropez lifestyle, a glass of wine is included with dinner most days in all of the phases except Phase 3. If you prefer not to have wine (or cocktails with equivalent calories), you can add another snack or have fruit juice.

Similarly, full-fat milk, yogurt, and cheese, which are often forbidden in diets, are included several times a week in most of the phases. In France, it's the quality of the cheese that's important—and people usually find that really excellent cheeses are so rich that just a small serving is enough to satisfy. I recommend sticking with full-fat dairy in small amounts so that you get the full benefit of the CLA in milk fats, but when you want to accelerate your weight loss, low-fat versions can help add flavor and nutrients without adding too many calories. Stay away from fat-free dairy, though, which has no benefits at all.

Instant Snacks or Meals

In addition to the recipes in Part 3, here are some ideas for super-quick snacks or meals. In a pinch, you can substitute one of these instant recipes, which are healthy and contain the right balance of omega-6 to omega-3 essential fatty acids while maintaining a low calorie count. Any of these options can serve as a quick snack. Or you can double the portion for a lunch and add 1 to 2 cups of raw vegetables such as carrots, bell peppers, or grape tomatoes. For dinners, serve a double portion with a small salad of dark greens and a simple vinaigrette made of 1 tablespoon olive or walnut oil and 1 or 2 tablespoons balsamic, red wine, rice, or herb vinegar. Watch the sodium content of seasoned vinegars; your vinegar should provide very little if any sodium. Finally, you'll see that many of these recipes call for low-fat yogurt; if you're not in a weight-loss phase, feel free to substitute full-fat yogurt to get the full benefits of the nutrients in milk fat.

BREAKFAST	Top a 6-ounce container of low-fat plain yogurt (Greek yogurt, if you can find it, is best) with 1 tablespoon of sliced olives, 2 tablespoons of either walnuts or pumpkin seeds (available unsalted and in bulk at many health food stores), and 1 tablespoon of ground flaxseed. (335 calories)
BREAKFAST	Sprinkle a 6-ounce container of low-fat plain yogurt with 2 tablespoons sliced almonds or chopped walnuts, 2 tablespoons oats, 1/2 cup fresh berries or 1/4 cup dried berries, and 1 tablespoon of honey. (349 calories)
BREAKFAST	Have 2 low-fat whole-grain frozen waffles (200 calories and at least 4 grams of fiber per two-waffle serving) topped with 1 cup sliced strawberries. (216 calories)
BREAKFAST	In a bowl, combine 6 ounces of low-fat lemon yogurt with 1/2 cup or 100 calories of your favorite whole grain cereal (with at least 4 grams of fiber per serving), 2 tablespoons slivered almonds, and 1 tablespoon ground flax meal. (400 calories)
BREAKFAST	Combine 2 cups of fruit (try a variety, such as berries, melon, and pomegranate) with 1/4 cup of nuts and 1/4 cup of unsweetened, dried fruit. (465 calories)
BREAKFAST	Cook 1/2 cup of dry oatmeal and top it with 1 cup chopped fruit and 2 tablespoons each of walnuts and sliced almonds and 1 tablespoon of maple syrup or honey. (464 calories)
LUNCH/ DINNER	Toast 1 whole wheat English muffin. Fill with 1/2 cup sliced red pepper and 3 ounces solid white tuna packed in water mixed with 2 tablespoons tahini or sesame butter. (440 calories)
LUNCH/ DINNER	Combine 1 cup canned broadbeans or fava beans, rinsed and drained, with 1/4 cup chopped Vidalia onion, 1/2 teaspoon minced garlic, 1 tablespoon extra virgin olive oil, 1 teaspoon lemon juice, and 1 tablespoon golden balsamic or rice vinegar. (231 calories)
LUNCH/ DINNER	In a bowl, mix 2 cups arugula, 1/4 sliced cucumber, 1/2 chopped bell pepper, and 5 chopped baby carrots. Sprinkle salad with 1 ounce or 1/3 cup pumpkin seeds and 4 anchovies. For the dressing, whisk together 1 tablespoon lemon juice or balsamic vinegar, 1 tablespoon of olive or walnut oil, and 1/2 teaspoon of chopped fresh dill. (456 calories)
LUNCH/ DINNER	Mix 2 ounces of solid white tuna packed in water with 2 teaspoons canola oil mayonnaise (rather than the usual kind, which is made with unhealthy vegetable oil). Cover a 1-ounce slice of walnut bread with your tuna salad. (231 calories)

LUNCH/ DINNER	Have 1/3 cup whole-milk ricotta cheese with 1/2 cup raspberries and 1 tablespoon each ground flaxseed, low-fat granola cereal, and chopped walnuts. (297 calories)
LUNCH/ DINNER	Fill an 8-inch whole wheat soft tortilla with a mixture of 1/4 cup corn, 1/4 cup canned precooked black beans (rinsed and drained), 1 tablespoon chopped fresh cilantro, 1/4 cup salsa, 1 teaspoon flaxseed or olive oil, 1 tablespoon lime juice, and 2 tablespoons cheddar cheese. (343 calories)
LUNCH/ DINNER	Open an 8-inch whole wheat pita and spread with 1 teaspoon of Dijon mustard. Add 3 ounces of diced chicken breast mixed with 1 tablespoon canola oil mayonnaise, a handful of baby spinach leaves, 2 slices tomato, pepper to taste, and 1/3 cup salsa. (459 calories)
LUNCH/ DINNER	Top 2 to 3 cups of dark leafy greens with 1/4 cup shredded carrots, 1 ounce or 1/4 cup total of walnuts, pumpkin seeds, and/or almonds, and 2 ounces canned tuna, salmon, sardines, or anchovies. (460 calories)
LUNCH/ DINNER	Combine 2 cups arugula, 1/2 cup chopped canned beets, 3 tablespoons walnuts, 1 tablespoon minced shallot, and 2 tablespoons feta cheese. For the dressing, whisk together 1 tablespoon minced shallot, 2 teaspoons flaxseed or olive oil, 1 tablespoon red wine or balsamic vinegar, and pepper to taste. (338 calories)
LUNCH/ DINNER	Top 2 cups baby spinach leaves with 1 chopped tomato, 2 ounces solid white tuna packed in water (drained), and 2 tablespoons sliced black olives. For the dressing, whisk together 1 tablespoon flaxseed or olive oil and 1 tablespoon red wine or balsamic vinegar. (289 calories)
LUNCH/ DINNER	Prepare 1 cup cooked whole wheat pasta, any shape. Toss cooked pasta with 2 teaspoons extra virgin olive oil, 1 teaspoon Parmesan cheese, 1/2 teaspoon of chopped fresh basil, 1 teaspoon minced garlic, 1 diced tomato, and 1/2 cup chopped red bell pepper. (297 calories)
LUNCH/ DINNER	Put 2 teaspoons of olive oil into a sauté pan and sear a 3-ounce salmon steak for approximately 2 minutes per side. Top with some chopped fresh dill and serve with 1 cup of steamed broccoli or spinach. Sprinkle with a dressing of 2 teaspoons of olive oil, a teaspoon of chopped fresh dill, and a squeeze of lemon. (396 calories)
LUNCH/ DINNER	Heat a skillet over low to medium heat with 1 tablespoon olive oil. Add 1 sliced red bell pepper, 1/4 cup each sliced mushrooms and chopped onion, 1 diced tomato, and a sprinkle of chopped fresh basil and oregano. Open and toast (if desired) 1 whole wheat roll, and top with the grilled vegetables. Serve with 1 sliced orange. (431 calories)

LUNCH/ DINNER	Combine 3 ounces diced roasted chicken breast, 1 diced tomato, 1 tablespoon each of canola oil mayonnaise and ground flaxseed, 1 teaspoon honey, 1 tablespoon red wine vinegar, and 2 teaspoons dried blueberries. Serve over 3 cups baby spinach leaves. (359 calories)
LUNCH/ DINNER	Prepare 1/2 cup cooked brown rice. In a saucepan heat 1 tablespoon olive oil and sauté 1/4 cup chopped red onion, 1/2 cup chopped red bell pepper, and 1 minced garlic clove for 4 minutes. Add 1/2 cup cooked brown rice, 1 teaspoon each fresh oregano and fresh parsley, and 1/2 teaspoon ground black pepper; heat for another 2 minutes. Remove from heat and add 1 1/2 ounces feta cheese. (386 calories)
LUNCH/ DINNER	In a bowl combine 2 cups shredded prepared cole slaw greens with 2 teaspoons canola oil mayonnaise, 1 teaspoon honey, 1 tablespoon balsamic vinegar, 4 ounces low-fat plain yogurt, and 2 teaspoons dried blueberries. Add 1 chopped apple and 4 tablespoons chopped walnuts. (473 calories)
LUNCH/ DINNER	In a bowl combine 3 ounces canned salmon with 2 tablespoons seasoned bread crumbs, 1 tablespoon canola oil mayonnaise, 1 tablespoon lemon juice, 1 egg white, 1 sliced spring onion, and 1/4 teaspoon Dijon mustard. Form into 2 patties, place on a nonstick baking dish, and bake at 350 degrees for 20 minutes. (339 calories)
SNACK	Smear a half-ounce slice of walnut bread with 1 tablespoon of pesto and top it with a half-ounce round of smoked salmon and 1 tomato slice. (109 calories)
SNACK	Smear a 1-ounce slice of walnut bread with 2 tablespoons each olive tapenade and chopped bell pepper, 2 anchovies, and 2 slices of tomato. (204 calories)
SNACK	Dip 10 baby carrots in 1 tablespoon olive tapenade. (110 calories)
SNACK	Dip 7 cherry tomatoes in 1 tablespoon olive tapenade. (97 calories)
SNACK	Have 1/2 cup red grapes with 1 tablespoon walnuts. (104 calories)
SNACK	Have 1 tablespoon dried blueberries or cranberries with 2 tablespoons chopped walnuts. (123 calories)
SNACK	Mix 3 1/2 ounces Greek yogurt with 1 tablespoon sliced black olives and 1 teaspoon slivered almonds. (141 calories)
SNACK	Mix 6 ounces low-fat plain yogurt with 2 teaspoons dried blueberries or raisins. (125 calories)

SNACK	Mix 1/2 cup low-fat plain yogurt with 1 tablespoon ground flaxseed. (141 calories)
SNACK	Dip 1 sliced orange bell pepper in dressing of 2 teaspoons flaxseed or olive oil, 1 teaspoon of chopped fresh herbs such as dill and basil, and 1 tablespoon red wine or balsamic vinegar. (111 calories)
SNACK	Have 1/4 cup whole-milk ricotta cheese mixed with 1 tablespoon apricot preserves and 1/4 teaspoon pure almond extract; stir well to combine. Add in 2 chopped fresh or canned (juice or water pack) apricots. (140 calories)
SNACK	In a blender, combine 1/3 cup 4% fat cottage cheese and 2 tablespoons chopped walnuts. Slice 1 orange bell pepper and dip in the spread. (194 calories)
DESSERT	Top a 6-ounce low-fat plain yogurt with 1/4 cup dried figs. (231 calories)
DESSERT	Have 1 1/2 cups of mixed berries, such as blueberries, raspberries, and blackberries. (98 calories)
DESSERT	Spread 1 apple with 1 tablespoon almond butter. (172 calories)
DESSERT	Have 1 sliced banana with 1 tablespoon chopped walnuts. (154 calories)
DESSERT	Slice 2 fresh peaches, and top with 1 tablespoon each chopped walnuts and slivered almonds. (178 calories)
DESSERT	Mix 6-ounces low-fat plain yogurt with 2 teaspoons cocoa powder and 1 teaspoon honey. (136 calories)
DESSERT	In a popsicle mold, freeze 1/2 cup natural pomegranate juice and 1/4 cup fresh squeezed orange juice to make a frozen fruit juice bar. (103 calories)
DESSERT	Slice a pear in half, remove core, and sprinkle with 1/2 teaspoon ground cinnamon, 1 teaspoon each brown sugar and slivered almonds, and 1 tablespoon wheat germ. Bake for approximately 12 minutes at 350 degrees F. (192 calories)
DESSERT	Chop 1 apple, top with 2 tablespoons slivered almonds, sprinkle with 1/4 teaspoon ground cinnamon and 1 teaspoon brown sugar. Heat in the microwave for 60 to 90 seconds. (188 calories)

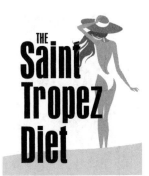

Introducing Good Fats and Fresh Ingredients

Week One—Approximately 1,600 Calories

This week you will learn a new way of eating, one that brings healthy fats into your diet mainly with fish, nuts, and fresh vegetables. Spend this week getting rid of your old habits and cleaning out your pantry of foods that are on the forbidden list. The time you spend shopping and cooking these new foods can be a celebration of a new lifestyle rather than a chore.

Remember that you don't need to cook everything on this suggested list. Leftovers can be used as substitutes throughout the week or you can use the quick snacks and meal suggestions from pages 84-87 when you are pressed for time.

Note that all of the meal suggestions are for one serving except where otherwise noted.

DAY ONE

BREAKFAST	In a bowl, combine 6 ounces of low-fat lemon yogurt with 1/2 cup or 100 calories of your favorite whole grain cereal (with at least 4 grams of fiber per serving), 2 tablespoons slivered almonds, and 1 tablespoon ground flax meal. (400 calories)
LUNCH	Carrot and Orange Soup (220 calories)
SNACK	2 Tomato and Walnut Bruschetta (94 calories)
DINNER	Salmon with Basil Aioli (608 calories)
	1 glass of wine (150 calories)
DESSERT	Orange Salad with Champagne (142 calories)

TOTAL CALORIES: 1,614

DAY TWO

BREAKFAST	Oat Bran Flax Muffin (258 calories)
LUNCH	Combine 3 ounces diced roasted chicken breast, 1 diced tomato, 1 tablespoon each of canola oil mayonnaise and ground flaxseed, 1 teaspoon honey, 1 tablespoon red wine vinegar, and 2 teaspoons dried blueberries. Serve over 3 cups baby spinach leaves. (359 calories)
SNACK	1/2 serving Carrot and Orange Soup (110 calories)
DINNER	Sea Bass with Ginger and Lime (306 calories)
	Wild Rice with Lentils (184 calories)
	1 glass of wine (150 calories)
DESSERT	Top a 6-ounce low-fat plain yogurt with 1/4 cup dried figs. (231 calories)

TOTAL CALORIES: 1,577

DAY THREE

BREAKFAST	Granola with Banana, Apple, and Walnut (325 calories)
LUNCH	Lentil Soup (184 calories)
	Tomatoes Provençal (130 calories)
SNACK	Have 1/4 cup whole-milk ricotta cheese mixed with 1 tablespoon apricot preserves and 1/4 teaspoon pure almond extract; stir well to combine. Add in 2 chopped fresh or canned (juice or water packed) apricots. (140 calories)
DINNER	Pork Roast with Figs (510 calories)
DESSERT	Oat Bran Flax Muffin (258 calories)

TOTAL CALORIES: 1,547

DAY FOUR

BREAKFAST	Whole Grain Bread with Laughing Cow Cheese, Pear, and Walnut (158 calories)
LUNCH	Heat a skillet over low to medium heat with 1 tablespoon olive oil. Add 1 sliced red bell pepper, 1/4 cup each sliced mushrooms and chopped onion, 1 diced tomato, and a sprinkle of chopped fresh basil and oregano. Open and toast (if desired) 1 whole wheat roll, and top with the grilled vegetables. Serve with 1 sliced orange. (431 calories)
SNACK	Dip 10 baby carrots in 1 tablespoon olive tapenade. (110 calories)
DINNER	Stuffed Eggplant (219 calories)
	Mesclun Greens with Goat Cheese Salad (444 calories)
DESSERT	Chop 1 apple, top with 2 tablespoons slivered almonds, sprinkle with 1/4 teaspoon ground cinnamon and 1 teaspoon brown sugar. Heat in the microwave for 60 to 90 seconds. (188 calories)

TOTAL CALORIES: 1,614

DAY FIVE

BREAKFAST	Granola with Banana, Apple, and Walnut (325 calories)
LUNCH	Melon with Figs and Prosciutto (233 calories)
SNACK	Dip 7 cherry tomatoes in 1 tablespoon olive tapenade. (97 calories)
DINNER	Stuffed Turkey Breast Italian Style (326 calories)
	2 servings of Green Beans with Tomatoes (200 calories)
	1 glass of wine (150 calories)
DESSERT	Spread 1 apple with 1 tablespoon almond butter. (172 calories)

TOTAL CALORIES: 1,503

DAY SIX

BREAKFAST	Omelet with Salmon and Asparagus (260 calories)
	Have 1 sliced banana with 1 tablespoon chopped walnuts. (154 calories)
LUNCH	Open an 8-inch whole wheat pita and spread with 1 teaspoon of Dijon mustard. Add 3 ounces of diced chicken breast mixed with 1 tablespoon canola oil mayonnaise, a handful of baby spinach leaves, 2 slices tomato, pepper to taste, and 1/3 cup salsa. (459 calories)
SNACK	1/2 serving of Melon with Figs and Prosciutto (116 calories)
DINNER	Red Snapper with Basil and Oregano, served with rice and tomato (394 calories)
	1 glass of wine (150 calories)
DESSERT	The Apostolos Crêpes with Chocolate and Nut Filling (114 calories for crêpe; 81 calories for filling)

TOTAL CALORIES: 1,622

DAY SEVEN

BREAKFAST	Rye Bread with Cream Cheese and Salmon (157 calories)
	2 cups red grapes (221 calories)
LUNCH	Combine 1 cup canned broadbeans or fava beans (rinsed and drained) with 1/4 cup chopped Vidalia onion, 1/2 teaspoon minced garlic, 1 tablespoon extra virgin olive oil, 1 teaspoon lemon juice, and 1 tablespoon golden balsamic or rice vinegar. (231 calories)
SNACK	Olive Paste and Red Bell Pepper Bruschetta (63 calories)
DINNER	Duck Breast with Berries (570 calories)
	1 glass of wine (150 calories)
DESSERT	Fig Compote with Yogurt (251 calories)

TOTAL CALORIES: 1,687

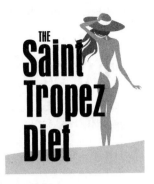

Balancing Diet and Lifestyle

Week Two—Approximately 1,450 Calories

Congratulate yourself for getting through the first week. You likely made some new choices and found that you weren't quite as hungry as you thought you would be. You also probably feel healthier; some people swear they can feel the toxins being removed from their bodies. Now is the time to add exercise to your regimen. No need to go crazy at the gym. In France, everyone walks everywhere, and that is the key to staying slim. Add 20 to 45 minutes of walking every day to your diet plan.

DAY EIGHT

BREAKFAST	Wheat Bran Flakes with Berries and Raisins (with 1% milk) (276 calories)
LUNCH	Pasta with Anchovies (447 calories)
SNACK	Have 1 tablespoon dried cranberries or blueberries with 2 tablespoons chopped walnuts. (123 calories)
DINNER	Mackerel with Mushrooms (457 calories)
DESSERT	Mix 6 ounces low-fat plain yogurt with 2 teaspoons cocoa powder and 1 teaspoon honey. (136 calories)

TOTAL CALORIES: 1,439

DAY NINE

BREAKFAST	Muesli with Dried Fruits and Nuts (293 calories)
LUNCH	In a bowl, combine 2 cups shredded prepared cole slaw greens with 2 teaspoons canola oil mayonnaise, 1 teaspoon honey, 1 tablespoon balsamic vinegar, 4 ounces low-fat plain yogurt, and 2 teaspoons dried blueberries. Add 1 chopped apple and 4 tablespoons chopped walnuts. (473 calories)
SNACK	Smear a half-ounce slice of walnut bread with 1 tablespoon of pesto and top it with a half-ounce round of smoked salmon and 1 tomato slice. (109 calories)
DINNER	Smoked Duck Salad with Raspberry Vinaigrette (410 calories)
DESSERT	Slice a pear in half, remove core, and sprinkle with 1/2 teaspoon ground cinnamon, 1 teaspoon each brown sugar and slivered almonds, and 1 tablespoon wheat germ. Bake for approximately 12 minutes at 350 degrees F. (192 calories)

TOTAL CALORIES: 1,477

DAY TEN

BREAKFAST	Whole Grain Bread with Almond Butter, Apricot Preserves, and Almonds (149 calories)
LUNCH	Fisherman Salad (409 calories)
SNACK	Dip 10 baby carrots in 1 tablespoon olive tapenade. (110 calories)
DINNER	Pasta with Sun-Dried Tomatoes and Artichokes (361 calories)
	1 glass of wine (150 calories)
DESSERT	Top a 6-ounce low-fat plain yogurt with 1/4 cup dried figs. (231 calories)

TOTAL CALORIES: 1,410

DAY ELEVEN

BREAKFAST	Whole Grain Bread with Almond Butter, Apricot Preserves, and Almond (149 calories)
	1 mango (115 calories)
LUNCH	Artichokes and Fava Beans Salad (403 calories)
SNACK	Have 1/2 cup red grapes with 1 tablespoon walnuts. (104 calories)
DINNER	Salmon and Fennel Papilotte (440 calories)
	1 glass of wine (150 calories)
DESSERT	Have 1 1/2 cups of mixed berries, such as blueberries, raspberries, and blackberries. (98 calories)

TOTAL CALORIES: 1,459

DAY TWELVE

BREAKFAST	Omelet Provence Style (232 calories)
LUNCH	Fisherman Salad (409 calories)
SNACK	Have 1 tablespoon dried cranberries or blueberries with 2 tablespoons chopped walnuts. (123 calories)
DINNER	Broil 5 ounces salmon with 1 tablespoon extra virgin olive oil. (378 calories) Swiss Chard Tagine (148 calories)
DESSERT	Marie's Oatmeal Cookies (123 calories) You may want to make a batch, freeze them, and pull one out as needed. Make sure it is properly sealed when frozen; otherwise, humidity would be a major problem. Defrost at room temperature for half an hour or so; do not microwave.

TOTAL CALORIES: 1,413

DAY THIRTEEN

BREAKFAST	Oatmeal with Almond, Apple, Apricot, and Mango (with 1% milk) (294 calories)
LUNCH	2 servings Beet and Fennel Soup (236 calories)
SNACK	Tomato Walnut Bruschetta (2 servings; 94 calories)
DINNER	Potato Parsnip Purée (158 calories)
	Swordfish with Walnuts (414 calories)
	1 glass of wine (150 calories)
DESSERT	Marie's Oatmeal Cookies (123 calories)

TOTAL CALORIES: 1,469

DAY FOURTEEN

BREAKFAST	Whole Grain Bread with Laughing Cow Cheese, Pear, and Walnuts (158 calories)
	1 mango (135 calories)
LUNCH	Lentil Salad (230 calories)
SNACK	Mix 6 ounces low-fat plain yogurt with 2 teaspoons dried blueberries or raisins. (125 calories)
DINNER	Dogfish with Spicy Red Wine Sauce (473 calories)
	Carrot Salad with Lemon (210 calories)
DESSERT	Chocolate and Nut Filling (81 calories)
	1/2 cup strawberries (23 calories)

TOTAL CALORIES: 1,435

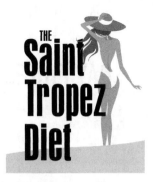

Reaching Your Ideal Weight

Weeks Three, Four, Five, and Six— Approximately 1,300 to 1,400 Calories

By restricting your calorie intake, increasing your exercise, and introducing omega-3 essential fatty acids into your diet, you've started to lose some weight. It may take several weeks to correct the long unbalanced ratio of omega-6 to omega-3 fatty acids. As that ratio changes, your skin tone, energy level, and body shape will change accordingly. Now it's time to step up all of these changes a little bit more so that you see results faster.

Note that while we've allowed for one glass of wine with dinner in most of the phases, in this phase we suggest that you forego alcohol altogether as an easy way to reduce your calorie intake. Also, avoiding alcohol will give you more energy and focus to increase your exercise intensity.

DAY FIFTEEN

BREAKFAST	Salmon and Asparagus Omelet (260 calories)
LUNCH	2 servings Pumpkin Soup (366 calories)
SNACK	Tomatoes Provence Style (130 calories)
DINNER	Sardines and Spinach au Gratin (432 calories)
DESSERT	Fruit Salad with Mint (165 calories)

TOTAL CALORIES: 1,353

DAY SIXTEEN

BREAKFAST	Oat Bran Flax Muffin (258 calories) You may want to make a batch, freeze them, and pull one out as needed. Defrost at room temperature or in the microwave for about 30 seconds on high.
LUNCH	Prepare 1 cup cooked whole wheat pasta, any shape. Toss cooked pasta with 2 teaspoons extra virgin olive oil, 1 teaspoon Parmesan cheese, 1/2 teaspoon chopped fresh basil, 1 teaspoon minced garlic, 1 diced tomato, and 1/2 cup chopped red bell pepper. (297 calories)
SNACK	Tomatoes Provençal (130 calories)
DINNER	Broiled Salmon with Dill (295 calories)
DESSERT	Baked Apples with Toasted Walnuts (156 calories)

TOTAL CALORIES: 1,182

DAY SEVENTEEN

BREAKFAST	Rye Bread with Cream Cheese and Salmon (157 calories)
LUNCH	Open an 8-inch whole wheat pita and spread with 1 teaspoon of Dijon mustard. Add 3 ounces of diced chicken breast mixed with 1 tablespoon canola oil mayonnaise, a handful of baby spinach leaves, 2 slices of tomato, pepper to taste, and 1/3 cup salsa. (459 calories)
SNACK	2 servings Olive Paste and Red Bell Pepper Bruschetta (126 calories)
DINNER	Hake with Leek Fondue (397 calories)
DESSERT	The Apostolos Crêpes with Chocolate and Nut Filling (114 calories for crêpes /81 calories for filling)

TOTAL CALORIES: 1,334

DAY EIGHTEEN

BREAKFAST	Wheat Bran Flakes with Berries (with 2% milk) (286 calories)
	1 small banana (65 calories)
LUNCH	Mushroom and Hazelnut Soup (293 calories)
SNACK	Have 1 tablespoon raisins and 2 tablespoons slivered almonds. (132 calories)
DINNER	Tuna with Balsamic Vinegar (319 calories)
DESSERT	The Apostolos Crêpes with Apple Filling (114 calories for crêpes /87 calories for filling)

TOTAL CALORIES: 1,296

DAY NINETEEN

BREAKFAST	Granola with Banana, Apple, and Walnut (325 calories)
LUNCH	Curly Endive Greek Style (392 calories)
SNACK	Dip 7 cherry tomatoes in 1 tablespoon olive tapenade. (97 calories)
DINNER	Sardines and Spinach au Gratin (432 calories)
DESSERT	Marie's Oatmeal Cookies (123 calories)

TOTAL CALORIES: 1,369

DAY TWENTY

BREAKFAST	Whole Grain Bread with Almond Butter, Apricot Preserves, and Almonds (149 calories)
LUNCH	1 cup canned lentil soup with less than 500 mg sodium per serving (store bought item) (110 calories)
	Beets with Walnuts (207 calories)
SNACK	Mix 1/2 cup low-fat plain yogurt with 1 tablespoon ground flaxseed. (141 calories)
DINNER	Chicken Breast with Garlic Cloves (497 calories)
	Tomatoes Provence Style (130 calories)
DESSERT	Have 1 sliced banana with 1 tablespoon chopped walnuts. (154 calories)

TOTAL CALORIES: 1,388

DAY TWENTY-ONE

BREAKFAST	Muesli with Dried Fruits and Nuts (293 calories)
LUNCH	Chicken Salad with Celery and Apple (304 calories)
SNACK	Tomatoes Provence Style (130 calories)
DINNER	Salmon with Orange Sauce (461 calories)
DESSERT	Marie's Oatmeal Cookies (123 calories)

TOTAL CALORIES: 1,311

DAY TWENTY-TWO

BREAKFAST	2 Buckwheat Crêpes with Cottage Cheese, Berries, and Kiwi (with topping) (382 calories)
LUNCH	Top 2 cups baby spinach leaves with 1 chopped tomato, 2 ounces solid white tuna packed in water (drained), and 2 tablespoons sliced black olives. For the dressing, whisk together 1 tablespoon flaxseed or olive oil and 1 tablespoon red wine or balsamic vinegar. (289 calories)
SNACK	Mix 1/2 cup low-fat plain yogurt with 1 tablespoon ground flaxseed. (141 calories)
DINNER	Tomato and Rice Soup (391 calories)
DESSERT	In a popsicle mold, freeze 1/2 cup pomegranate juice and 1/4 cup fresh-squeezed orange juice to make a frozen fruit juice bar. (103 calories)

TOTAL CALORIES: 1,316

DAY TWENTY-THREE

BREAKFAST	Oat Bran Flax Muffin (259 calories)
LUNCH	Tomato and Rice Soup (391 calories)
SNACK	Have 1 tablespoon dried cranberries or blue- berries with 2 tablespoons chopped walnuts. (123 calories)
DINNER	Pork Loin with Tomato Coulis (333 calories) Risotto with Olives (137 calories)
DESSERT	Orange Salad with Champagne (142 calories)

TOTAL CALORIES: 1,385

DAY TWENTY-FOUR

BREAKFAST	2 Buckwheat Crêpes with Cottage Cheese, Berries, and Kiwi (without topping) (276 calories)
LUNCH	Toast 1 whole wheat English muffin. Fill with 1/2 cup sliced red bell pepper and 3 ounces solid white tuna packed in water mixed with 2 tablespoons tahini or sesame butter. (440 calories)
SNACK	Have 1/2 cup cubed honeydew topped with 1 tablespoon chopped walnuts. (113 calories)
DINNER	Cod Fish with Ratatouille and Feta Cheese (354 calories)
DESSERT	Mix 6 ounces low-fat plain yogurt with 2 teaspoons cocoa powder and 1 teaspoon honey. (136 calories)

TOTAL CALORIES: 1,319

DAY TWENTY-FIVE

BREAKFAST	Oatmeal with Almond, Apricot, Apple, and Mango (with 2% milk) (329 calories)
LUNCH	Cod Fish with Ratatouille and Feta Cheese (354 calories)
SNACK	Dip 1 sliced orange bell pepper in dressing of 2 teaspoons flaxseed or olive oil, 1 teaspoon of chopped fresh herbs (such as dill and basil), and 1 tablespoon red wine or balsamic vinegar. (111 calories)
DINNER	Chicken Salad with Celery and Apple (304 calories)
	100 calories of whole grain cracker with at least 2 grams of fiber (100 calories)
DESSERT	Marie's Oatmeal Cookies (123 calories)

TOTAL CALORIES: 1,321

DAY TWENTY-SIX

BREAKFAST	Muesli with Dried Fruits and Nuts (293 calories)
LUNCH	Combine 2 cups arugula, 1/2 cup chopped canned beets, 3 tablespoons walnuts, 1 tablespoon minced shallot, and 2 tablespoons feta cheese. For the dressing, whisk together 1 tablespoon minced shallot, 2 teaspoons flaxseed or olive oil, 1 tablespoon red wine or balsamic vinegar, and pepper to taste. (338 calories)
SNACK	Mix 3 1/2 ounces Greek yogurt with 1 tablespoon sliced black olives and 1 teaspoon slivered almonds. (141 calories)
DINNER	Trout with Almonds (476 calories)
DESSERT	In a popsicle mold, freeze 1/2 cup natural pomegranate juice and 1/4 cup fresh squeezed orange juice to make a frozen fruit juice bar. (103 calories)

TOTAL CALORIES: 1,351

DAY TWENTY-SEVEN

BREAKFAST	Rye Bread with Cream Cheese and Salmon (157 calories)
	1 apple (70 calories)
LUNCH	Chicken Salad with Celery and Apple (304 calories)
SNACK	Smear a half-ounce slice of walnut bread with 1 tablespoon of pesto, and top it with a half-ounce round of smoked salmon and 1 tomato slice. (109 calories)
DINNER	Tuna Basque Style (443 calories)
DESSERT	Have 2 sliced fresh peaches topped with 1 tablespoon each chopped walnuts and slivered almonds. (178 calories)

TOTAL CALORIES: 1,261

DAY TWENTY-EIGHT

BREAKFAST	Omelet Provence Style (232 calories)
LUNCH	Mesclun Greens with Goat Cheese (444 calories)
SNACK	Smear a half-ounce slice of walnut bread with 1 tablespoon of pesto, and top it with a half-ounce round of smoked salmon and 1 tomato slice. (109 calories)
DINNER	Salmon and Fennel Papilotte (440 calories)
DESSERT	Marie's Oatmeal Cookies (123 calories)

TOTAL CALORIES: 1,348

DAY TWENTY-NINE

BREAKFAST	Salmon and Asparagus Omelet (260 calories)
	1 apple (70 calories)
LUNCH	Prepare 1/2 cup cooked brown rice. In a saucepan, heat 1 tablespoon olive oil and sauté 1/4 cup chopped red onion, 1/2 cup chopped red bell pepper, and 1 minced garlic clove for 4 minutes. Add 1/2 cup cooked brown rice, 1 teaspoon each fresh oregano and fresh parsley, and 1/2 teaspoon ground black pepper; heat for another 2 minutes. Remove from heat and add 1 1/2 ounces feta cheese. (386 calories)
SNACK	Mix 6 ounces low-fat plain yogurt with 2 teaspoons dried blueberries. (125 calories)
DINNER	Mushroom and Hazelnut Soup (293 calories)
	Have 1/2 cup red grapes with 1 tablespoon walnuts. (104 calories)
DESSERT	In a popsicle mold, freeze 1/2 cup natural pomegranate juice and 1/4 cup fresh squeezed orange juice to make a frozen fruit juice bar. (103 calories)

TOTAL CALORIES: 1,341

DAY THIRTY

BREAKFAST	Oat Bran Flax Muffin (258 calories)
LUNCH	In a bowl, combine 2 cups shredded prepared cole slaw greens with 2 teaspoons canola oil mayonnaise, 1 teaspoon honey, 1 tablespoon balsamic vinegar, 4 ounces low-fat plain yogurt, and 2 teaspoons dried blueberries. Add 1 chopped apple and 4 tablespoons chopped walnuts. (473 calories)
SNACK	Smear a half-ounce slice of walnut bread with 1 tablespoon of pesto, and top it with a half-ounce round of smoked salmon and 1 tomato slice. (109 calories)
DINNER	Broiled Salmon with Dill (295 calories)
DESSERT	Fruit Salad with Mint (165 calories)

TOTAL CALORIES: 1,300

DAY THIRTY-ONE

BREAKFAST	Rye Bread with Cream Cheese and Salmon (157 calories)
LUNCH	Open an 8-inch whole wheat pita and spread with 1 teaspoon of Dijon mustard. Add 3 ounces of diced chicken breast mixed with 1 tablespoon canola oil mayonnaise, a handful of baby spinach leaves, 2 slices tomato, pepper to taste, and 1/3 cup salsa. (446 calories)
SNACK	Smear a half-ounce slice of walnut bread with 1 tablespoon of pesto, and top it with a half-ounce round of smoked salmon and 1 tomato slice. (109 calories)
DINNER	Stuffed Bell Peppers (200 calories)
	Spinach with Pine Nuts and Raisins (187 calories)
DESSERT	Fruit Salad with Mint (165 calories)

TOTAL CALORIES: 1,627

DAY THIRTY-TWO

BREAKFAST	Wheat Bran Flakes with Berries (with 2% milk) (286 calories)
LUNCH	In a bowl, mix 2 cups arugula, 1/4 sliced cucumber, 1/2 chopped bell pepper, and 5 chopped baby carrots. Sprinkle salad with 1 ounce or 1/3 cup pumpkin seeds and 4 anchovies. For the dressing, whisk together 1 tablespoon lemon juice or balsamic vinegar, 1 tablespoon of olive or walnut oil, and 1/2 teaspoon of chopped fresh dill. (456 calories)
SNACK	Have 1/2 cup red grapes with 1 tablespoon walnuts. (104 calories)
DINNER	Tuna with Balsamic Vinegar (319 calories)
DESSERT	The Apostolos Crêpes with Chocolate and Nut Filling (114 calories for crêpes /81 calories for filling)

TOTAL CALORIES: 1,360

DAY THIRTY-THREE

BREAKFAST	Granola with Banana, Apple, and Walnut (325 calories)
LUNCH	White Bean Stew (461 calories)
SNACK	Dip 7 cherry tomatoes in 1 tablespoon olive tapenade. (97 calories)
DINNER	Chicken Salad with Celery and Apple (304 calories)
DESSERT	Marie's Oatmeal Cookies (123 calories)

TOTAL CALORIES: 1,310

DAY THIRTY-FOUR

BREAKFAST	Whole Grain Bread with Almond Butter, Apricot Preserves, and Almonds (149 calories)
LUNCH	In a bowl, combine 3 ounces canned salmon with 2 tablespoons seasoned bread crumbs, 1 tablespoon canola oil mayonnaise, 1 tablespoon lemon juice, 1 egg white, 1 sliced spring onion, and 1/4 teaspoon Dijon mustard. Form into 2 patties, place on a nonstick baking dish and bake at 350 degrees for 20 minutes. (339 calories)
SNACK	Mix 1/2 cup low-fat plain yogurt with 1 tablespoon ground flaxseed. (141 calories)
DINNER	Niçoise Salad (560 calories)
DESSERT	In a popsicle mold, freeze 1/2 cup natural pomegranate juice and 1/4 cup fresh squeezed orange juice to make a frozen fruit juice bar. (103 calories)

TOTAL CALORIES: 1,292

DAY THIRTY-FIVE

BREAKFAST	Muesli with Dried Fruits and Nuts (293 calories)
LUNCH	Top 2 cups baby spinach leaves with 1 chopped tomato, 2 ounces solid white tuna packed in water (drained), and 2 tablespoons sliced black olives. For the dressing, whisk together 1 tablespoon flaxseed or olive oil and 1 tablespoon red wine or balsamic vinegar. (289 calories)
SNACK	Dip 7 cherry tomatoes in 1 tablespoon olive tapenade. (97 calories)
DINNER	Salmon with Orange Sauce (461 calories)
DESSERT	Marie's Oatmeal Cookies (123 calories)

TOTAL CALORIES: 1,263

DAY THIRTY-SIX

BREAKFAST	Omelet Provence Style (232 calories)
LUNCH	Tomato and Rice Soup (391 calories)
SNACK	Mix 1/2 cup low-fat plain yogurt with 1 table-spoon ground flaxseed. (141 calories)
DINNER	Artichokes and Fava Beans Salad (403 calories)
DESSERT	In a popsicle mold, freeze 1/2 cup natural pomegranate juice and 1/4 cup fresh squeezed orange juice to make a frozen fruit juice bar. (103 calories)

TOTAL CALORIES: 1,270

DAY THIRTY-SEVEN

BREAKFAST	Oat Bran Flax Muffin (259 calories)
LUNCH	Fill an 8-inch whole wheat soft tortilla with a mixture of 1/4 cup corn, 1/4 cup canned precooked black beans (rinsed and drained), 1 tablespoon chopped fresh cilantro, 1/4 cup salsa, 1 teaspoon flaxseed or olive oil, 1 tablespoon lime juice, and 2 tablespoons cheddar cheese. (343 calories)
SNACK	Have 2 tablespoons sunflower seeds and 1 tablespoon dried blueberries. (127 calories)
DINNER	Fish Soup (486 calories)
DESSERT	Slice 2 fresh peaches and top with 1 tablespoon each chopped walnuts and slivered almonds. (178 calories)

TOTAL CALORIES: 1,393

DAY THIRTY-EIGHT

BREAKFAST	Have 2 low-fat whole-grain frozen waffles (200 calories and at least 4 grams of fiber per 2-waffle serving) topped with 1 cup sliced strawberries. (216 calories)
LUNCH	Toast 1 whole wheat English muffin. Fill with 1/2 cup sliced red bell pepper and 3 ounces solid white tuna packed in water mixed with 2 tablespoons tahini or sesame butter. (440 calories)
SNACK	Have 1/2 cup cubed honeydew topped with 1 tablespoon chopped walnuts. (113 calories)
DINNER	Trout with Almonds (476 calories)
DESSERT	Mix 6 ounces low-fat plain yogurt with 2 teaspoons cocoa powder and 1 teaspoon honey. (136 calories)

TOTAL CALORIES: 1,381

DAY THIRTY-NINE

BREAKFAST	Oatmeal with Almond, Apricot, Apple, and Mango (with 2% milk) (329 calories)
LUNCH	Have 3 cups shredded romaine lettuce with 3 tablespoons sliced black olives, 3 tablespoons feta cheese, 1 diced tomato, and 1 diced red pepper. Whisk together 1 tablespoon walnut oil with 1 tablespoon white balsamic vinegar for the dressing. (310 calories)
SNACK	Dip 1 sliced orange bell pepper in dressing of 2 teaspoons flaxseed or olive oil, 1 teaspoon of chopped fresh herbs (such as dill and basil), and 1 tablespoon red wine or balsamic vinegar. (111 calories)
DINNER	Chickpea, Tomato, and Rice Soup (391 calories)
DESSERT	Marie's Oatmeal Cookies (123 calories)

TOTAL CALORIES: 1,264

DAY FORTY

BREAKFAST	Omelet Provence Style (232 calories)
LUNCH	Combine 2 cups arugula, 1/2 cup chopped canned beets, 3 tablespoons walnuts, 1 table-spoon minced shallot, and 2 tablespoons feta cheese. For the dressing, whisk together 1 tablespoon minced shallot, 2 teaspoons flaxseed or olive oil, 1 tablespoon red wine or balsamic vinegar, and pepper to taste. (338 calories)
SNACK	Mix 3 1/2 ounces Greek yogurt with 1 table-spoon sliced black olives and 1 teaspoon slivered almonds. (141 calories)
DINNER	Trout with Almonds (476 calories)
DESSERT	In a popsicle mold, freeze 1/2 cup natural pomegranate juice and 1/4 cup fresh squeezed orange juice to make a frozen fruit juice bar. (103 calories)

TOTAL CALORIES: 1,290

DAY FORTY-ONE

BREAKFAST	2 servings Rye Bread with Cream Cheese and Salmon (314 calories)
LUNCH	Chicken Salad with Celery and Apple (304 calories)
SNACK	Smear a half-ounce slice of walnut bread with 1 tablespoon of pesto, and top it with a half-ounce round of smoked salmon and 1 tomato slice. (109 calories)
DINNER	Lentil Salad (230 calories)
	Pumpkin Soup (183 calories)
DESSERT	Have 2 sliced fresh peaches topped with 1 tablespoon each chopped walnuts and slivered almonds. (178 calories)

TOTAL CALORIES: 1,318

DAY FORTY-TWO

BREAKFAST	Granola with Banana, Apple, and Walnut (325 calories)
LUNCH	Prepare 1/2 cup cooked brown rice. In a saucepan, heat 1 tablespoon olive oil and sautée 1/4 cup chopped red onion, 1/2 cup chopped red bell pepper, and 1 minced garlic clove for 4 minutes. Add 1/2 cup cooked brown rice, 1 teaspoon fresh oregano and fresh parsley, and 1/2 teaspoon ground black pepper; heat for another 2 minutes. Remove from heat and add 1 1/2 ounces feta cheese. (386 calories)
SNACK	Smear a half-ounce slice of walnut bread with 1 tablespoon of pesto, and top it with a half-ounce round of smoked salmon and 1 tomato slice. (109 calories)
DINNER	Salmon and Fennel Papilotte (440 calories)
DESSERT	Marie's Oatmeal Cookies (123 calories)

TOTAL CALORIES: 1,383

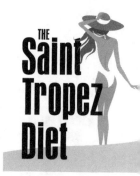

THE
Saint
Tropez
Diet

Maintaining a Healthy Lifestyle

Weeks Seven and Eight—
Approximately 1,500 to 1,600 Calories

Once you've reached a healthy weight, or if you're feeling too hungry
or restricted on Phase 3, it's time for maintenance. By now, we hope
you've become a convert to the Saint-Tropez way of eating. After all,
who wouldn't love to be eating fresh, gourmet meals and enjoying fine
wine and decadent desserts—and still fitting into the tiniest bikini—
all year round? Remember, it's easy to eat the way the French do. Just
eat more fresh foods and fewer packaged foods; more fish and fewer
red meat; more fruits and vegetables and fewer cakes and cookies. And
take the time to enjoy your meals—and drink to your health!

DAY FORTY-THREE

BREAKFAST	Wheat Bran Flakes with Berries and Raisins (with 1% milk) (276 calories) 1 pomegranate (104 calories)
LUNCH	Chicken Salad with Celery and Apple (304 calories)
SNACK	Dip 10 baby carrots in 1 tablespoon olive tapenade. (110 calories)
DINNER	Mackerel with Mushrooms (457 calories) Drizzle 2 sliced tomatoes with 1 1/2 tablespoons olive oil, and sprinkle with ground black pepper. (229 calories)
DESSERT	In a popsicle mold, freeze 1/2 cup natural pomegranate juice and 1/4 cup fresh squeezed orange juice to make a frozen fruit juice bar. (103 calories)

TOTAL CALORIES: 1,583

DAY FORTY-FOUR

BREAKFAST	Muesli with Dried Fruits and Nuts (293 calories)
LUNCH	In a bowl, mix 2 cups arugula, 1/4 sliced cucumber, 1/2 chopped bell pepper, and 5 chopped baby carrots. Sprinkle salad with 1 ounce or 1/3 cup pumpkin seeds and 4 anchovies. For the dressing, whisk together 1 tablespoon lemon juice or balsamic vinegar, 1 tablespoon of olive or walnut oil, and 1/2 teaspoon of chopped fresh dill. (456 calories)
SNACK	Smear a half-ounce slice of walnut bread with 1 tablespoon of pesto, and top it with a half-ounce round of smoked salmon and 1 tomato slice. (109 calories)
DINNER	Smoked Duck Salad with Raspberry Vinaigrette (410 calories)
	Apple and Walnut Bruschetta (88 calories)
DESSERT	Slice a pear in half, remove core, and sprinkle with 1/2 teaspoon ground cinnamon, 1 teaspoon each brown sugar and slivered almonds, and 1 tablespoon wheat germ. Bake for approximately 12 minutes at 350 degrees F. (192 calories)

TOTAL CALORIES: 1,548

DAY FORTY-FIVE

BREAKFAST	Top a 6-ounce container of low-fat plain yogurt (Greek yogurt, if you can find it, is best) with 1 tablespoon of sliced olives, 2 tablespoons of either walnuts or pumpkin seeds (available unsalted and in bulk at many health food stores), and 1 tablespoon of ground flaxseed. (335 calories)
LUNCH	Fisherman Salad (409 calories)
SNACK	Dip 7 cherry tomatoes in 1 tablespoon olive tapenade. (110 calories)
DINNER	Pasta with Sun-Dried Tomatoes and Artichokes (361 calories)
	1 glass of wine (150 calories)
DESSERT	Figs Compote with Yogurt (251 calories)

TOTAL CALORIES: 1,616

DAY FORTY-SIX

BREAKFAST	2 servings Whole Grain Bread with Almond Butter, Apricot Preserves, and Almond (298 calories)
	1 mango (115 calories)
LUNCH	Artichokes and Fava Beans Salad (403 calories)
SNACK	Have 1/2 cup red grapes with 1 tablespoon walnuts. (104 calories)
DINNER	Eggplant au Gratin (371 calories)
	1 glass of wine (150 calories)
DESSERT	Strawberries with Spicy Red Wine Sauce (144 calories)

TOTAL CALORIES: 1,585

DAY FORTY-SEVEN

BREAKFAST	Omelet Provence Style (232 calories)
	Chop 1 apple, top with 2 tablespoons slivered almonds, sprinkle with 1/4 teaspoon ground cinnamon, and 1 teaspoon brown sugar. Heat in the microwave for 60 to 90 seconds. (188 calories)
LUNCH	Toast 1 whole wheat English muffin. Fill with 1/2 cup sliced red pepper and 3 ounces solid white tuna packed in water mixed with 2 tablespoons tahini or sesame butter. (440 calories)
SNACK	Have 1 tablespoon dried cranberries or blueberries with 2 tablespoons chopped walnuts. (123 calories)
DINNER	Broil 4 ounces salmon with 1 tablespoon extra virgin olive oil. (308 calories)
	Beets with Walnuts (207 calories)
DESSERT	In a popsicle mold, freeze 1/2 cup natural pomegranate juice and 1/3 cup fresh squeezed orange juice to make a frozen fruit juice bar. (103 calories)

TOTAL CALORIES: 1,601

DAY FORTY-EIGHT

BREAKFAST	Oatmeal with Almond, Apple, Apricot, and Mango (with 1% milk) (294 calories)
	1 orange and one 1-ounce slice mozzarella cheese (132 calories)
LUNCH	Open an 8-inch whole wheat pita and spread with 1 teaspoon of Dijon mustard. Add 3 ounces of diced chicken breast mixed with 1 tablespoon canola oil mayonnaise, a handful of baby spinach leaves, 2 slices tomato, pepper to taste, and 1/3 cup salsa. (459 calories)
SNACK	Have 1/4 cup whole-milk ricotta cheese mixed with 1 tablespoon apricot preserves and 1/4 teaspoon pure almond extract; stir well to combine. Add in 2 chopped fresh or canned (juice or water packed) apricots. (140 calories)
DINNER	Sole Fillets with White Beans Velouté (401 calories)
DESSERT	Mix 6 ounces low-fat plain yogurt with 2 teaspoons cocoa powder and 1 teaspoon honey. (136 calories)

TOTAL CALORIES: 1,562

DAY FORTY-NINE

BREAKFAST	2 servings Whole Grain Bread with Laughing Cow Cheese, Pear, and Walnuts (316 calories)
	1 apple (70 calories)
LUNCH	In a bowl, combine 2 cups shredded prepared cole slaw greens with 2 teaspoons canola oil mayonnaise, 1 teaspoon honey, 1 tablespoon balsamic vinegar, 4 ounces low-fat plain yogurt, and 2 teaspoons dried blueberries. Add 1 chopped apple and 4 tablespoons chopped walnuts. (473 calories)
SNACK	Mix 6 ounces low-fat plain yogurt with 2 teaspoons dried blueberries or raisins. (125 calories)
DINNER	Sea Bream with Almonds and Edible Flowers (396 calories)
	1 glass of wine (150 calories)
DESSERT	In a popsicle mold, freeze 1/2 cup natural pomegranate juice and 1/4 cup fresh squeezed orange juice to make a frozen fruit juice bar. (103 calories)

TOTAL CALORIES: 1,633

DAY FIFTY

BREAKFAST	Wheat Bran Flakes with Berries and Raisins (with 1% milk) (276 calories)
LUNCH	Pasta with Anchovies (447 calories)
SNACK	Smear a half-ounce slice of walnut bread with 1 tablespoon of pesto, and top it with a half-ounce round of smoked salmon and 1 tomato slice. (109 calories)
DINNER	Mackerel with Mushrooms (457 calories)
	1 cup cubed cantaloupe with 2 tablespoons chopped walnuts (158 calories)
DESSERT	In a popsicle mold, freeze 1/2 cup natural pomegranate juice and 1/4 cup fresh squeezed orange juice to make a frozen fruit juice bar. (103 calories)

TOTAL CALORIES: 1,550

DAY FIFTY-ONE

BREAKFAST	Muesli with Dried Fruits and Nuts (293 calories)
	1 cup whole milk (146 calories)
LUNCH	Fill an 8-inch whole wheat soft tortilla with a mixture of 1/4 cup corn, 1/4 cup canned precooked black beans (rinsed and drained), 1 tablespoon chopped fresh cilantro, 1/4 cup salsa, 1 teaspoon flaxseed or olive oil, 1 tablespoon lime juice, and 2 tablespoons cheddar cheese. (343 calories)
SNACK	Smear a half-ounce slice of walnut bread with 1 tablespoon of pesto, and top it with a half-ounce round of smoked salmon and 1 tomato slice. (109 calories)
DINNER	Trout with Almonds (476 calories)
DESSERT	Slice a pear in half, remove core, and sprinkle with 1/2 teaspoon ground cinnamon, 1 teaspoon each brown sugar and slivered almonds, and 1 tablespoon wheat germ. Bake for approximately 12 minutes at 350 degrees F. (192 calories)

TOTAL CALORIES: 1,559

DAY FIFTY-TWO

BREAKFAST	Whole Grain Bread with Almond Butter, Apricot Preserves, and Almonds (149 calories)
	1 pear (96 calories)
LUNCH	Toast 1 whole wheat English muffin. Fill with 1/2 cup sliced red pepper and 3 ounces solid white tuna packed in water mixed with 2 tablespoons tahini or sesame butter. (440 calories)
SNACK	Dip 10 baby carrots in 1 tablespoon olive tapenade. (110 calories)
DINNER	Lamb Chops with Herbs (363 calories)
	1 glass of wine (150 calories)
DESSERT	Oat Bran Flax Muffin (258 calories)

TOTAL CALORIES: 1,460

DAY FIFTY-THREE

BREAKFAST	Omelet Provence Style (232 calories)
	Spread 1 apple with 1 tablespoon almond butter. (172 calories)
LUNCH	Have 3 cups shredded romaine lettuce with 3 tablespoons sliced black olives, 3 tablespoons feta cheese, 1 diced tomato, and 1 diced red bell pepper. Whisk together 1 tablespoon walnut oil with 1 tablespoon white balsamic vinegar for the dressing. (310 calories)
SNACK	Have 1/2 cup red grapes with 1 tablespoon walnuts. (104 calories)
DINNER	Salmon and Fennel Papilotte (440 calories)
	1 glass of wine (150 calories)
DESSERT	In a popsicle mold, freeze 1/2 cup natural pomegranate juice and 1/4 cup fresh squeezed orange juice to make a frozen fruit juice bar. (103 calories)

TOTAL CALORIES: **1,511**

DAY FIFTY-FOUR

BREAKFAST	Oat Bran Flax Muffin (258 calories)
	Have 1 sliced banana with 1 tablespoon chopped walnuts. (154 calories)
LUNCH	In a bowl, mix 2 cups arugula, 1/4 sliced cucumber, 1/2 chopped bell pepper, and 5 chopped baby carrots. Sprinkle salad with 1 ounce or 1/3 cup pumpkin seeds and 4 anchovies. For the dressing, whisk together 1 tablespoon lemon juice or balsamic vinegar, 1 tablespoon olive or walnut oil, and 1/2 teaspoon chopped fresh dill. (456 calories)
SNACK	Have 1 tablespoon dried cranberries or blueberries with 2 tablespoons chopped walnuts. (123 calories)
DINNER	Artichokes and Fava Beans Salad (403 calories)
DESSERT	Mix 6 ounces low-fat plain yogurt with 2 teaspoons cocoa powder and 1 teaspoon honey. (136 calories)

TOTAL CALORIES: 1,530

DAY FIFTY-FIVE

BREAKFAST	Oatmeal with Almond, Apple, Apricot, and Mango (with 1% millk) (294 calories)
	One 1-ounce slice cheddar cheese (114 calories)
LUNCH	Combine 2 cups arugula, 1/2 cup chopped canned beets, 3 tablespoons walnuts, 1 table-spoon minced shallot, and 2 tablespoons feta cheese. For the dressing, whisk together 1 table-spoon minced shallot, 2 teaspoons flaxseed or olive oil, 1 tablespoon red wine or balsamic vinegar, and pepper to taste. (338 calories)
SNACK	Have 1 tablespoon dried cranberries with 2 ta-blespoons chopped walnuts. (123 calories)
DINNER	Swordfish with Walnuts (414 calories)
	1 glass of wine (150 calories)
DESSERT	Fruit Salad with Mint (165 calories)

TOTAL CALORIES: 1,598

DAY FIFTY-SIX

BREAKFAST	Wheat Bran Flakes with Berries and Raisins (with 1% milk) (276 calories)
	24 almonds (about 1/4 cup) (211 calories)
	1 apple (72 calories)
LUNCH	Combine 1 cup canned broadbeans or fava beans (rinsed and drained) with 1/4 cup chopped Vidalia onion, 1/2 teaspoon minced garlic, 1 tablespoon extra virgin olive oil, 1 teaspoon lemon juice, and 1 tablespoon golden balsamic or rice vinegar. (231 calories)
SNACK	Mix 6 ounces low-fat plain yogurt with 2 teaspoons dried blueberries or raisins. (125 calories)
DINNER	Salmon with Orange Sauce (461 calories)
DESSERT	Fruit Salad with Mint (165 calories)

TOTAL CALORIES: 1,541

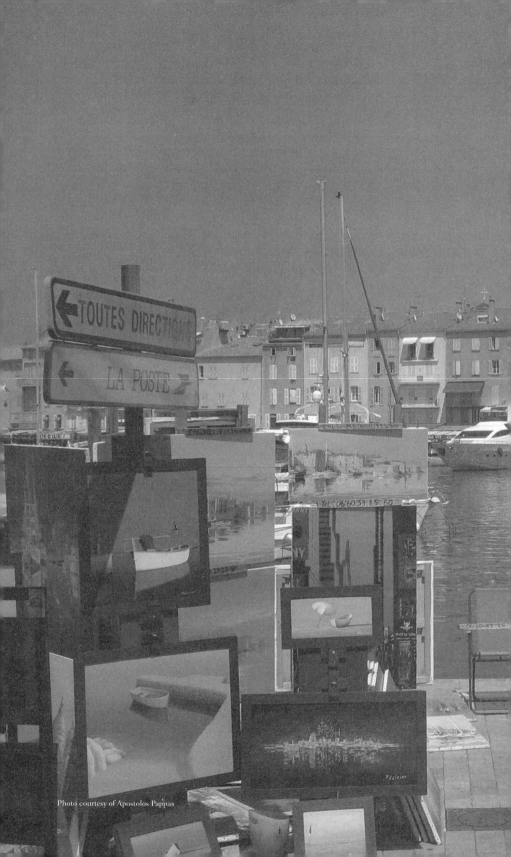

Recipes for the Saint-Tropez Diet

In Saint-Tropez, eating well means cooking well. The recipes that follow will help you to do just that—cook your way to a leaner, healthier body. If you are a novice in the kitchen, don't be alarmed by the elegant French titles of these recipes because they are generally easy to prepare. We've organized the recipes from easy (marked "e") to medium "m") to complex ("c"). Those that require steps beyond chopping or dicing have clear, easy-to-follow instructions. In the end you will have meals that are easy, flavorful, and healthy.

As you grow more experienced, you'll find many recipes to try, including several by prominent French chefs. These are the same dishes they serve in the top restaurants in and around Saint-Tropez. Master these, and you will be bringing a bit of Provence into your own kitchen.

When you first work with the recipes that follow, you'll want to stick closely to the instructions and pay particular attention to the portion sizes so that you are not sabotaging your diet with excess calories. Each recipe contains detailed nutritional information, as well as tips for preserving leftovers.

We've also included wine suggestions for the entrees. But keep in mind, these are just our personal preferences. As you grow accustomed to this new way of eating, feel free to experiment with new combinations. The goal, ultimately, is not just to lose weight, but to begin your own culinary adventure as if you lived on the French Riviera. Bon Appetit!

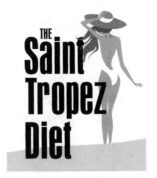

Breakfasts

Omelette au Saumon et Asperges
(SALMON AND ASPARAGUS OMELET)

Heat the oil in a nonstick pan over medium heat. Add the onions and sauté until translucent. Add the garlic, asparagus, lemon juice, and sauté for 2 minutes. Spread the vegetables evenly on the bottom of the pan.

In a bowl, beat the eggs, milk, and herbs, and season to taste. Add the egg mixture to the asparagus and let the eggs set. Add the smoked salmon, reduce heat, and continue to cook for 2 to 3 minutes. Fold over in half, cook for another minute, and serve immediately.

8 eggs
2 teaspoons canola oil
1 tablespoon milk
6 ounces smoked salmon
8 asparagus spears, cooked
2 ounces onions, diced (about 1/2 small onion)
1 garlic clove, minced
1 teaspoon fresh chives, minced
1 teaspoon fresh dill, minced
2 tablespoons fresh parsley, minced
1 teaspoon lemon juice
Salt and pepper to taste

SERVING SIZE: 1/4 recipe

PER SERVING: 260 Cal (56% from Fat, 38% from Protein, 6% from Carb); 24 g Protein; 16 g Tot Fat; 4 g Sat Fat; 7 g Mono Fat; 4 g Carb; 1 g Fiber; 2 g Sugar; 97 mg Calcium; 4 mg Iron; 503 mg Sodium; 501 mg Cholesterol

YIELD: 4 servings

Rye Bread with Cream Cheese and Salmon

Spread the cream cheese over the bread. Add the smoked salmon, sprinkle with a little lemon juice, and serve immediately.

1 slice rye bread
3/4 ounce cream cheese
3/4 ounce smoked salmon
A few drops lemon juice

Option: You may add a little fresh dill and lemon juice to the cream cheese. The idea is to bring more flavors into the cream cheese. I often prepare cream and cheese this way and stock it for a few days ready to go. It is more convenient, tates better, and is cheaper than buying flavored cream cheese. You will still need a few drops of lemon juice on top of the salmon to bring out its flavor.

SERVING SIZE: 1 slice

TOTAL RECIPE: 157 Cal (33% from Fat, 23% from Protein, 44% from Carb); 9 g Protein; 6 g Tot Fat; 3 g Sat Fat; 2 g Mono Fat; 17 g Carb; 2 g Fiber; 0 g Sugar; 50 mg Calcium; 1 mg Iron; 441 mg Sodium; 17 mg Cholesterol

YIELD: 1 serving

Whole Grain Bread with Laughing Cow Cheese, Pear, and Walnut

Spread the cheese over the bread. Layer the pear slices on top, sprinkle with walnuts, and serve immediately.

1 slice whole grain bread

3/4 ounce low-fat Laughing Cow or other low-calorie spreadable cheese

2 ounces pear slices

1/2 teaspoon walnut, chopped

SERVING SIZE: 1 slice

TOTAL RECIPE: 158 Cal (26% from Fat, 15% from Protein, 59% from Carb); 6 g Protein; 5 g Tot Fat; 2 g Sat Fat; 1 g Mono Fat; 24 g Carb; 4 g Fiber; 9 g Sugar; 79 mg Calcium; 1 mg Iron; 174 mg Sodium; 11 mg Cholesterol

YIELD: 1 serving

Whole Grain Bread with Almond Butter, Apricot Preserves, and Almond

Spread the almond butter over the bread. Add the apricot preserves, sprinkle the almonds, and serve immediately.

1 slice whole grain bread

1 teaspoon almond butter

1 teaspoon apricot preserves

1 teaspoon almonds

SERVING SIZE: 1 slice

PER SERVING: 149 Cal (34% from Fat, 12% from Protein, 54% from Carb); 5 g Protein; 6 g Tot Fat; 1 g Sat Fat; 3 g Mono Fat; 21 g Carb; 3 g Fiber; 7 g Sugar; 51 mg Calcium; 1 mg Iron; 159 mg Sodium; 0 mg Cholesterol

YIELD: 1 serving

Granola with Banana, Apple, and Walnut

Mix the granola with the milk. Add the banana, apples, walnuts, and serve immediately.

SERVING SIZE: 1/2 cup

PER SERVING: 325 Cal (18% from Fat, 11% from Protein, 71% from Carb); 9 g Protein; 7 g Tot Fat; 2 g Sat Fat; 2 g Mono Fat; 60 g Carb; 5 g Fiber; 28 g Sugar; 171 mg Calcium; 2 mg Iron; 185 mg Sodium; 10 mg Cholesterol

YIELD: 1 serving

1/2 cup granola
1/2 cup milk
1 ounce banana, sliced
(about 1/4 small banana)
1 ounce apple, diced
(about a 1/4 medium apple)
1 teaspoon walnuts, chopped

Oatmeal with Almond, Apricot, Apple, and Mango

Place the oatmeal in a bowl, add the boiling liquid, and mix well. Mix in the sunflower seeds, almonds, dried apricot, apple, and mango. Serve immediately.

1/2 cup oatmeal

1 cup water or milk

1 teaspoon sunflower seeds

1 teaspoon almonds

1 teaspoon dried apricot, diced

1 ounce apple, diced (about a 1/4 medium apple)

1 ounce mango, diced (about a 1/4 medium mango)

SERVING SIZE: 1/2 cup oatmeal

PER SERVING: 191 Cal (13% from Fat, 11% from Protein, 76% from Carb); 6 g Protein; 3 g Tot Fat; 0 g Sat Fat; 1 g Mono Fat; 40 g Carb; 6 g Fiber; 8 g Sugar; 31 mg Calcium; 1 mg Iron; 8 mg Sodium; 0 mg Cholesterol (water)

PER SERVING: 294 Cal (15% from Fat, 18% from Protein, 67% from Carb); 14 g Protein; 5 g Tot Fat; 2 g Sat Fat; 2 g Mono Fat; 52 g Carb; 6 g Fiber; 21 g Sugar; 316 mg Calcium; 2 mg Iron; 111 mg Sodium; 12 mg Cholesterol (1% milk)

PER SERVING: 329 Cal (20% from Fat, 18% from Protein, 62% from Carb); 15 g Protein; 8 g Tot Fat; 3 g Sat Fat; 3 g Mono Fat; 53 g Carb; 6 g Fiber; 21 g Sugar; 378 mg Calcium; 2 mg Iron; 148 mg Sodium; 20 mg Cholesterol (2% milk)

YIELD: 1 serving

Muesli with Dried Fruits and Nuts

In a bowl, mix the cereal with the yogurt. If too thick, add a little milk to thin out. Top with the mixed dried berries and raisins, almonds, and walnuts. Serve immediately.

SERVING SIZE: 1/2 cup muesli

PER SERVING: 293 Cal (22% from Fat, 15% from Protein, 63% from Carb); 12 g Protein; 7 g Tot Fat; 2 g Sat Fat; 3 g Mono Fat; 49 g Carb; 5 g Fiber; 22 g Sugar; 262 mg Calcium; 4 mg Iron; 217 mg Sodium; 7 mg Cholesterol

YIELD: 1 serving

1/2 cup muesli cereal

1/2 cup yogurt

1/2 ounce mixed dried
    berries and raisins
    (about 2 tablespoons)

1 teaspoon almonds,
    slivered or sliced

1 teaspoon walnuts,
    chopped

Milk (regular or 2%)
    (optional)

Wheat Bran Flakes with Berries and Raisins

In a bowl, mix the cereal with the milk. Top with the berries, raisins, and flaxseed.

1 cup wheat bran flakes

1/2 cup milk

1/4 cup mixed fresh berries

1 tablespoon raisins

1 teaspoon flaxseed

SERVING SIZE: 1 cup wheat bran flakes

PER SERVING: 276 Cal (9% from Fat, 15% from Protein, 76% from Carb); 11 g Protein; 3 g Tot Fat; 1 g Sat Fat; 1 g Mono Fat; 58 g Carb; 8 g Fiber; 17 g Sugar; 180 mg Calcium; 3 mg Iron; 59 mg Sodium; 6 mg Cholesterol (1% milk)

PER SERVING: 286 Cal (12% from Fat, 14% from Protein, 74% from Carb); 11 g Protein; 4 g Tot Fat; 2 g Sat Fat; 1 g Mono Fat; 58 g Carb; 8 g Fiber; 16 g Sugar; 178 mg Calcium; 3 mg Iron; 55 mg Sodium; 10 mg Cholesterol (2% milk)

YIELD: 1 serving

Omelette Provençale
(OMELET PROVENCE STYLE)

Make a small X incision on the top and bottom of the tomatoes. Blanch the tomatoes for 20 seconds. Place in ice-cold water to stop the cooking process. Peel, seed, and dice the tomatoes.

Heat the oil in a nonstick pan over medium heat. Add the onions and sauté until translucent. Add the garlic, bell peppers, and cook for 3 minutes. Add the tomatoes and sauté quickly. Add the spinach, herbs, and season to taste. Spread the vegetables evenly over the bottom of the pan.

In a bowl, beat the eggs and milk and season to taste. Add the egg mixture to the vegetables and let the eggs set. Reduce heat and continue to cook for 2 to 3 minutes. Fold in half, cook for another minute, and serve immediately.

8 eggs
1 tablespoon milk
2 teaspoons olive oil
2 ounces onions, diced (about 1/2 small onion)
6 ounces tomatoes (about 1 large tomato)
3 garlic cloves, minced
6 ounces bell peppers
   (about 1 large bell pepper)
6 ounces cooked spinach, chopped
   (about 2/3 cup cooked spinach)
2 tablespoons fresh salad herbs, minced
Salt and pepper to taste

SERVING SIZE: 1/4 recipe

PER SERVING: 232 Cal (55% from Fat, 30% from Protein, 15% from Carb); 17 g Protein; 14 g Tot Fat; 4 g Sat Fat; 6 g Mono Fat; 9 g Carb; 3 g Fiber; 3 g Sugar; 148 mg Calcium; 4 mg Iron; 203 mg Sodium; 491 mg Cholesterol

YIELD: 4 servings

Oat Bran Flax Muffin

Preheat the oven to 350 degrees F.

Blend the flours, flaxseed meal, brown sugar, baking soda, baking powder, salt, cinnamon, and ginger in a mixing bowl. Mix in the carrots, apples, walnuts, and berries-raisins blend. Add the canola oil, vanilla, eggs, milk, and mix until well incorporated. Fill muffin pan and bake for 20 to 25 minutes.

Note: This recipe can be quite laxative.

SERVING SIZE: 1 muffin

PER SERVING: 258 Cal (36% from Fat, 8% from Protein, 56% from Carb); 6 g Protein; 11 g Tot Fat; 1 g Sat Fat; 4 g Mono Fat; 38 g Carb; 4 g Fiber; 19 g Sugar; 82 mg Calcium; 2 mg Iron; 280 mg Sodium; 41 mg Cholesterol

YIELD: 12 servings

1 cup unbleached all-purpose flour
1/2 cup oat bran flour
1/2 cup flaxseed meal
1/2 cup brown sugar
1 1/2 teaspoons baking soda
1 teaspoon baking powder
1/4 teaspoon salt
1 1/2 tablespoons ground cinnamon
1 teaspoon ground ginger
1 1/4 cups carrots, shredded
10 ounces apples, diced small
3/4 cup walnuts, chopped
3/4 cup berries-raisins blend
1/4 cup canola oil
1 teaspoon vanilla extract
2 eggs, mixed
1/2 cup milk

Buckwheat Crêpes with Cottage Cheese, Berries, and Kiwi

Place the flour in a bowl. Blend in the eggs, oil, honey, vanilla, and salt. Slowly whisk in the milk. Let the batter rest for 30 minutes. Before use, add a little water to thin out.

Heat a nonstick pan or crêpe pan over medium heat. Soak a small piece of paper towel with 1 teaspoon grapeseed oil and swirl the greased towel quickly over the pan. Add enough batter and swirl to cover the entire bottom. Cook until golden brown and turn over. Cook until golden brown. Repeat this process until all the crêpe batter is used.

Fill each crêpe with about 3/4 ounce cottage cheese and roll up. Top with 3 tablespoons berries and 1 tablespoon maple syrup each.

1/2 cup all-purpose flour
1/2 cup buckwheat flour
2 eggs
1 tablespoon honey
2 tablespoons grapeseed oil
1 cup milk
1 teaspoon vanilla extract
Pinch salt
8 ounces cottage cheese
2 cups fresh berries
Grapeseed oil for greasing the pan
10 tablespoons maple syrup

SERVING SIZE: 1 crêpe plus 3 tablespoons berries and 1 tablespoon maple syrup

PER SERVING: 138 Cal (33% from Fat, 21% from Protein, 46% from Carb); 7 g Protein; 5 g Tot Fat; 1 g Sat Fat; 2 g Mono Fat; 16 g Carb; 2 g Fiber; 5 g Sugar; 65 mg Calcium; 1 mg Iron; 124 mg Sodium; 53 mg Cholesterol (1 filled crêpe)

PER SERVING: 191 Cal (24% from Fat, 15% from Protein, 61% from Carb); 7 g Protein; 5 g Tot Fat; 1 g Sat Fat; 2 g Mono Fat; 30 g Carb; 3 g Fiber; 16 g Sugar; 80 mg Calcium; 1 mg Iron; 125 mg Sodium; 53 mg Cholesterol (1 filled crêpe with 3 tablespoons berries and 1 tablespoon maple syrup)

YIELD: 10 servings

Fish Entrees

Pâtes aux Anchois
(PASTA WITH ANCHOVIES)

| 12 ounces whole grain spaghetti |
| 1 tablespoon olive oil |

Preheat the oven to 425 degrees F.

Cook the spaghetti according to package directions. Strain, add a little bit of the oil from the anchovy can, mix, and set aside for later use.

Heat the oil in a nonstick pan over high heat. Add the onions and sauté until translucent. Add the garlic, bell peppers, and continue to cook for 3 minutes over medium heat. Add the sun-dried tomatoes, capers, olives, dried red pepper flakes, and anchovies. Sprinkle pepper and continue to cook for 2 to 3 minutes. Mix in the pasta, herbs, and Parmesan cheese. Adjust seasoning and serve immediately.

This dish may be refrigerated up to 2 days.

This dish may be frozen up to 1 month.

1 cup sun-dried tomatoes, julienned

2 ounces anchovy fillets (canned), chopped

4 ounces onions, diced small (about 1 small onion)

1 tablespoon garlic cloves, minced

6 ounces green bell peppers, diced medium (about 1 large green bell pepper)

1 tablespoon capers, drained

2 ounces pitted kalamata olives

1 teaspoon dried red pepper flakes

1/4 cup fresh basil, chopped

3 tablespoons fresh parsley, chopped

2 tablespoons Parmesan cheese

Salt and pepper to taste

Wine Suggestion: A young and sharp white (such as Chardonnay from Northern Italy or Chile or Assyrtiko from Santorini) or rosé (from Provence). You can even try a red such as a young Rioja or Primitivo.

SERVING SIZE: 1/4 recipe

PER SERVING: 447 Cal (17% from Fat, 17% from Protein, 66% from Carb); 21 g Protein; 9 g Tot Fat; 2 g Sat Fat; 5 g Mono Fat; 79 g Carb; 4 g Fiber; 7 g Sugar; 153 mg Calcium; 6 mg Iron; 1049 mg Sodium; 15 mg Cholesterol

YIELD: 4 Servings

Saumon Grillé à l'Aneth
(Broiled Salmon with Dill)

Four 5-ounce salmon fillets

1 tablespoon olive oil

4 to 5 fresh dill branches, minced

Salt and pepper to taste

Preheat the broiler. Place the fillets on a greased pan. Brush olive oil over the fish. Sprinkle with pepper and dill. Broil 3 to 4 minutes. Turn over, brush with oil, sprinkle with pepper and dill, and continue to broil for 3 to 4 minutes or until the salmon flesh starts to flake. Transfer to a serving platter and sprinkle salt to taste.

This fish goes well with the Marinated Vegetables with Lemon (see page 274) and lemon wedges.

The fish may be refrigerated up to 2 days and frozen up to 1 month.

Wine Suggestion: Salmon an be paired with either white or red. Keep your best white bottle for it (such as Montrachet, Chablis Grand Cru, California Chardonnay, Alsacian Riesling, or Rheingau Kabinett) or pair it with red (like a young Merlot or Pinot Noir).

Serving Size: One 5-ounce salmon fillet

Per Serving: 295 Cal (57% from Fat, 39% from Protein, 4% from Carb); 29 g Protein; 19 g Tot Fat; 4 g Sat Fat; 8 g Mono Fat; 3 g Carb; 1 g Fiber; 0 g Sugar; 34 mg Calcium; 1 mg Iron; 85 mg Sodium; 84 mg Cholesterol (fish)

Yield: 4 servings

Thon au Vinaigre de Balsamique
(Tuna with Balsamic Vinegar)

Preheat the broiler.

Blanch the pearl onions in boiling water for 2 minutes. Strain, cool, and peel.

Heat 1 tablespoon olive oil in a skillet over medium heat. Add the pearl onions and brown. Add the vinegar, shallot, garlic, honey, and reduce by half.

Meanwhile place the fillets on a greased baking pan. Brush olive oil over the fish and sprinkle with pepper. Broil for 3 to 4 minutes. Turn over, brush with oil, and continue to cook for a few minutes or until the flesh starts to flake.

Place the fish in a serving platter and sprinkle a little salt. Add the pearl onions and pour over the sauce.

Four 5-ounce tuna fillets
2 tablespoons olive oil
1 1/2 cups balsamic vinegar
1 shallot, minced
1 large garlic clove, minced
1 tablespoon honey
1 cup pearl onions
2 tablespoons fresh parsley, minced
Salt and pepper to taste

This recipe goes well with the Broccoli with Pistachio Vinaigrette (see page 273).

The fish and vegetables may be refrigerated separately up to 2 days.

The fish and vegetables may be frozen separately up to 1 month.

Wine Suggestion: Chardonnay from California or Australia or a mild Pinot Noir.

SERVING SIZE: One 5-ounce tuna fillet

PER SERVING: 319 Cal (38% from Fat, 42% from Protein, 20% from Carb); 34 g Protein; 14 g Tot Fat; 3 g Sat Fat; 7 g Mono Fat; 16 g Carb; 1 g Fiber; 12 g Sugar; 33 mg Calcium; 2 mg Iron; 60 mg Sodium; 54 mg Cholesterol (fish)

YIELD: 4 servings

Truite à la Grecque
(TROUT GREEK STYLE)

Preheat the broiler.

For the fish: In a bowl, blend the dry herbs. Place the trout on a flat surface and open them. Sprinkle some salt, pepper, and a large pinch of the dry herbs on each trout. Add 1 teaspoon fresh parley and 1 teaspoon fresh mint. Sprinkle with a little lemon juice and close the trout. Place the trout on a greased baking pan. Sprinkle olive oil over the trout. Broil for 3 to 4 minutes. Carefully turn over, brush with oil, and continue to broil for another 3 to 4 minutes.

Four 5-ounce trout, whole
1 tablespoon olive oil
1/4 teaspoon dried thyme
1/4 teaspoon dried coriander
1/4 teaspoon dried marjoram
1/4 teaspoon dried rosemary
1/4 teaspoon dried basil
4 teaspoons fresh parsley, minced
4 teaspoons fresh mint, minced
1 lemon
Salt and pepper to taste

This recipe goes well with Spinach with Pine Nuts and Raisins (see page 263).

The fish and vegetables may be refrigerated separately up to 2 days.

Not recommended for freezing.

Wine Suggestion: Rhoditis or Robola from Greece or a mild German Riesling.

SERVING SIZE: One 5-ounce trout

PER SERVING: 247 Cal (47% from Fat, 48% from Protein, 5% from Carb); 30 g Protein; 13 g Tot Fat; 2 g Sat Fat; 7 g Mono Fat; 3 g Carb; 2 g Fiber; 0 g Sugar; 90 mg Calcium; 3 mg Iron; 77 mg Sodium; 82 mg Cholesterol (fish)

YIELD: 4 servings

Truite aux Amandes
(Trout with Almonds)

Preheat the oven to 400 degrees F.

For the vegetables: Bring to a boil enough water to cover the green beans. Add 1 teaspoon of salt. Add the green beans and bring to a boil again. Reduce heat and simmer until tender. Strain and transfer to a serving plate, sprinkle with lemon juice, and season to taste.

For the fish: Cover a baking sheet with parchment paper. Spread the sliced almonds and bake until golden brown. Remove from the oven and set aside.

Sprinkle salt and pepper to taste inside the trout. Heat 1 tablespoon olive oil in a nonstick pan over medium heat. Add the trout and cook for 3 minutes. Carefully turn over and continue to cook 3 to 4 minutes or until cooked through.

Place the trout in a serving platter and sprinkle with the almonds. Cover to keep warm. Place the remaining oil, lemon juice, and parsley into a pan. Bring to a boil and pour over the trout. Serve immediately with green beans and lemon wedges.

The fish and vegetables may be refrigerated separately up to 2 days.

Not recommended for freezing.

Wine Suggestion: Meursault, mature Chardonnay, or late harvest Riesling.

FOR THE FISH:
Four 5-ounce trout, whole
4 tablespoons olive oil
2 ounces sliced almonds
1 tablespoon lemon juice
1 tablespoon fresh parsley
1 lemon, quartered
Salt and pepper to taste

FOR THE VEGETABLES:
24 ounces green beans
1 lemon
Salt and pepper to taste

SERVING SIZE: One 5-ounce trout

PER SERVING: 476 Cal (54% from Fat, 29% from Protein, 17% from Carb); 36 g Protein; 30 g Tot Fat; 4 g Sat Fat; 19 g Mono Fat; 21 g Carb; 10 g Fiber; 3 g Sugar; 194 mg Calcium; 5 mg Iron; 87 mg Sodium; 82 mg Cholesterol

YIELD: 4 servings

Morue Charbonnière au Miel et Thym
(SABLEFISH WITH HONEY AND THYME)

Combine the honey, wine, stock, and thyme in a saucepan. Bring to boil over high heat. Reduce heat and reduce to 3/4 cup. If necessary, thicken with a little cornstarch mixed with water.

Sprinkle pepper over the fillets. Heat the oil in a nonstick pan over medium heat. Add the fillets and brown. Carefully turn over, sprinkle with lemon juice, and continue to cook for 3 to 4 minutes. Pour in the prepared sauce, parsley, and bring to a boil. Adjust seasonings.

Four 5-ounce sablefish fillets
1 tablespoon olive oil
1/4 cup honey
1/4 cup white Muscat
1 cup vegetable stock
   (low-sodium)
1 teaspoon fresh thyme, minced
1 tablespoon lemon juice
2 tablespoons fresh
   parsley, minced
Cornstarch and water
Salt and pepper to taste

This dish goes well with the Orange-Glazed Carrots (see page 260).

The fish and vegetables may be refrigerated separately up to 2 days.

The fish and vegetables may be frozen separately up to 1 month.

Chef's Tip: The amount of cornstarch and water mixture may vary depending on the amount of water rendered by the fish and the reduction process. To obtain the right thickness for a sauce: Dip a spoon in the sauce, turn it over, and make a line across with your finger. Tilt the spoon. If the sauce does not run over the line, it is the perfect thickness. If it does, you need to thicken with a little cornstarch and water mixture. After adding them, you will need to bring the sauce to a boil. Also, if it gets too thick, just add a little liquid to thin out.

Wine Suggestion: A white Muscat.

SERVING SIZE: One 5-ounce sablefish fillet

PER SERVING: 369 Cal (11% from Fat, 28% from Protein, 61% from Carb); 27 g Protein; 5 g Tot Fat; 1 g Sat Fat; 3 g Mono Fat; 59 g Carb; 0 g Fiber; 54 g Sugar; 57 mg Calcium; 1 mg Iron; 146 mg Sodium; 61 mg Cholesterol (fish)

YIELD: 4 servings

Espadon aux Câpres
(SWORDFISH WITH CAPERS)

Preheat the oven to 375 degrees F.

For the fish: Heat the oil in an ovenproof nonstick pan over high heat. Add the swordfish and brown on both sides. Sprinkle pepper over the steaks, add a little lemon juice, and place in the oven. Cook until the flesh starts to flake. Remove the fish from the pan and place on a serving platter. Cover with aluminum foil to keep warm.

Deglaze the fish pan with the wine over high heat. To deglaze, add a liquid (such as wine, stock, or water) and swirl to dissolve cooked particles on the bottom or side of the pan. It is an important step in order to include all the extracted flavors, resulting in a more flavorful sauce. Add the garlic, 1 tablespoon capers, a little capers juice, and the remaining lemon juice. Reduce by half, strain, crushing the capers, and return the sauce to the pan. Add the stock and bring to a boil. Thicken with a little cornstarch mixed with water. Add the chives, remaining capers, and adjust seasonings. Bring to a boil, pour over the fillets, and serve immediately.

For the vegetables: Preheat a steamer. Add the carrots and cook covered until you reach almost the desired tenderness. Add the broccoli and continue to cook for 1 to 2 minutes. Transfer to a serving plate, season to taste, and add the lemon wedges.

FOR THE FISH:
Four 5-ounce swordfish steaks
2 teaspoons olive oil
3 tablespoons capers
1 tablespoon garlic cloves, minced
1/2 cup Sauvignon Blanc wine
1/2 cup fish or vegetable stock or
    combination (low-sodium)
1 lemon, juiced
Cornstarch with a little water
1 tablespoon chives, minced
Salt and pepper to taste

FOR THE VEGETABLES:
1 pound baby carrots
1 pound broccoli florets
1 lemon, quartered
Salt and pepper to taste

The fish and vegetables may be refrigerated separately up to 2 days.

The fish and vegetables may be frozen separately up to 1 month.

Chef's Tip: The amount of cornstarch and water mixture may vary depending on the amount of water rendered by the fish and the reduction process. To obtain the right thickness for a sauce: Dip a spoon in the sauce, turn it over, and make a line across with your finger. Tilt the spoon. If the sauce does not run over the line, it is the perfect thickness. If it does, you need to thicken with a little cornstarch and water mixture. After adding them, you will need to bring the sauce to a boil. Also, if it gets too thick, just add a little liquid to thin out.

Chef's Secret: If a fishy sauce is not your favorite, use vegetable stock. My favorite is to use half fish and half vegetable stock.

Wine Suggestion: Sauvignon Blanc.

SERVING SIZE: One 5-ounce swordfish steak

PER SERVING: 305 Cal (27% from Fat, 45% from Protein, 28% from Carb); 33 g Protein; 9 g Tot Fat; 2 g Sat Fat; 4 g Mono Fat; 21 g Carb; 4 g Fiber; 6 g Sugar; 115 mg Calcium; 3 mg Iron; 435 mg Sodium; 55 mg Cholesterol

YIELD: 4 servings

Colin à la Fondue de Poireaux
(HAKE WITH LEEK FONDUE)

FOR THE FISH:

Four 5-ounce hake fish fillets

1 1/2 pounds leeks (about 5 medium leeks)

1 tablespoon canola oil

1/4 cup vegetable stock (low-sodium)

1 tablespoon Dijon mustard

2 tablespoons crème fraiche

2 tablespoons lemon juice

2 tablespoons fresh chives, minced

Salt and pepper to taste

FOR THE VEGETABLES:

1 pound potatoes, peeled and quartered
  (about 3 medium potatoes)

1 pound yellow squash, chopped into 1-inch
  lengths (about 3 large yellow squash)

Salt and pepper to taste

Cut and discard the green part of the leeks. Cut the white part in half and julienne. Wash well to remove any dirt and pat dry.

Heat the oil in a large sauté pan over high heat. Add the leeks and sauté for 2 minutes. Add the stock and spread the leek on the bottom of the pan. Place the fish on top and sprinkle with pepper. Cover and cook for 20 minutes over low heat.

Meanwhile, preheat the steamer. Add the potatoes and cook for 15 minutes. Add the squash and continue to cook for 5 minutes.

Remove the fish and set aside in a serving platter. Cover with aluminum foil to keep warm. Add the lemon juice, mustard, crème fraiche, and chives to the leeks. Mix well, adjust seasonings, and reduce for 2 minutes. Pour the sauce over the fish and serve immediately with the vegetables.

The fish and vegetables may be refrigerated separately up to 2 days.

The fish and vegetables may be frozen separately up to 1 month.

Wine Suggestion: Sauvignon Blanc.

SERVING SIZE: One 5-ounce hake fillet

PER SERVING: 397 Cal (12% from Fat, 36% from Protein, 51% from Carb); 36 g Protein; 5 g Tot Fat; 1 g Sat Fat; 2 g Mono Fat; 52 g Carb; 10 g Fiber; 6 g Sugar; 115 mg Calcium; 4 mg Iron; 148 mg Sodium; 61 mg Cholesterol

YIELD: 4 servings

Gratin de Sardines aux Epinards
(SARDINES AND SPINACH AU GRATIN)

Remove the head and bones from the sardines (this can be done at the fish market). Rinse the sardines inside and out, and carefully dry with paper towels.

Blanch the spinach for 2 minutes in boiling salted water. Strain, pressing hard to remove any excess water. Chop and set aside.

Heat 1 tablespoon olive oil in a sauté pan over high heat. Add the onions and sauté until translucent. Add the garlic, spinach, and cook for 2 minutes mixing constantly. Add the crème fraiche, parsley, nutmeg, and season to taste. Reduce heat and continue to cook for 3 to 4 minutes.

Preheat the oven to 375 degrees F.

Sprinkle pepper inside each sardine and spread a little spinach mixture. Close without pressing. Place the remaining spinach mixture on the bottom of a greased baking dish. Add the sardines and sprinkle the remaining olive oil over the sardines. Spread the bread crumbs and bake for 15 to 20 minutes. Serve immediately with the lemon wedges.

The fish and vegetables may be refrigerated separately up to 2 days.

Wine Suggestion: Very dry white, such as Chardonnay, Assyrtiko from Santorini, Muscadet, or Vinho Verde.

Four 5-ounce fresh sardines
2 pounds fresh spinach, washed
3 tablespoons olive oil
6 ounces onions, diced small (about 1 medium onion)
1 tablespoon garlic cloves, minced
4 tablespoons crème fraiche
1 bunch fresh parsley, minced
2 tablespoons bread crumbs
2 pinches nutmeg
1 lemon, quartered
Salt and pepper to taste

SERVING SIZE: One 5-ounce sardine

PER SERVING: 432 Cal (50% from Fat, 32% from Protein, 17% from Carb); 36 g Protein; 25 g Tot Fat; 5 g Sat Fat; 13 g Mono Fat; 20 g Carb; 8 g Fiber; 5 g Sugar; 484 mg Calcium; 7 mg Iron; 333 mg Sodium; 86 mg Cholesterol

YIELD: 4 servings

Harengs Farcis aux Pommes de Terre et Oignons
(STUFFED HERRINGS WITH POTATOES AND ONIONS)

Place the potatoes into a pan and cover with water. Add 1 teaspoon salt and bring to a boil over high heat. Reduce heat and simmer for 15 minutes. When barely cooked, strain, and let cool. Peel and slice the potatoes.

Preheat the oven to 400 degrees F.

Heat the canola oil in a nonstick pan over high heat. Add the onions and slightly brown. Add the garlic and continue to cook for 1 minute. Remove from heat and cool down.

Four 4-ounce herrings
1 teaspoon canola oil
2 teaspoons olive oil
8 ounces onions, sliced (about 1 large onion)
Four 3-ounce red potatoes (about 4 small red potatoes)
1 tablespoon garlic cloves, minced
1 bunch fresh parsley, minced
Dash white wine vinegar
Salt and pepper to taste

Place each herring on one aluminum foil. Open the herrings and sprinkle with a little pepper. Equally divide the potatoes and onions among the herrings. Sprinkle with olive oil and parsley. Close the foils tight and place in a baking dish. Bake for 25 to 30 minutes. Serve immediately with a dash of white wine vinegar.

The fish and vegetables may be refrigerated separately up to 2 days.

Not recommended for freezing.

Wine Suggestion: Dry acidic Greek or Northern Italian white or white Burgundy (Bourgogne Aligoté) or Muscadet.

SERVING SIZE: One 4-ounce herring

PER SERVING: 471 Cal (34% from Fat, 27% from Protein, 39% from Carb); 32 g Protein; 18 g Tot Fat; 4 g Sat Fat; 8 g Mono Fat; 46 g Carb; 8 g Fiber; 4 g Sugar; 141 mg Calcium; 8 mg Iron; 1061 mg Sodium; 93 mg Cholesterol

YIELD: 4 servings

Lotte à la Provençale
(MONKFISH PROVENCE STYLE)

Four 5-ounce monkfish fillets
1 tablespoon olive oil
2 pounds tomatoes
  (about 6 large tomatoes)
8 ounces onions, sliced
  (about 1 large onion)
8 ounces green bell peppers, seeded,
  ribs removed, and sliced
  (about 1 large green bell pepper)
8 ounces yellow bell peppers, seeded,
  ribs removed, and sliced
  (about 1 large yellow bell pepper)
2 tablespoons garlic cloves, minced
2 pinches herbs de Provence
1 bunch fresh basil, shredded
1/2 cup brown rice
Salt and pepper to taste

Make a small X incision on the top and bottom of the tomatoes. Blanch the tomatoes for 20 seconds. Remove and place in ice-cold water to stop the cooking process. Peel, seed, and slice the tomatoes.

Cook the rice according to package instructions.

Heat the oil in a large pan over high heat. Add the monkfish and brown. Turn over and cook for 2 minutes. Remove the fish and set aside on a plate.

Deglaze the pan with a little water. To deglaze, add a liquid (such as wine, stock, or water) and swirl to dissolve cooked particles on the bottom or side of the pan. Add the onions and cook for 2 minutes. Add the garlic, tomatoes, bell peppers, herbs de Provence, and sauté for 2 minutes. Slide in the fish fillets, cover, and cook for 20 minutes over low heat. Remove the fillets and set aside in a platter. Cover with aluminum foil to keep warm. Mix the basil into the vegetables and season to taste. Pour over the fish and serve immediately with the rice.

The fish and rice may be refrigerated separately up to 2 days.

The fish and rice may be frozen separately up to 1 month.

Wine Suggestion: A Provence rosé, a Pinot Noir, or a mild Merlot.

SERVING SIZE: ONE 5-ounce monkfish fillet

PER SERVING: 328 Cal (19% from Fat, 31% from Protein, 50% from Carb); 26 g Protein; 7 g Tot Fat; 1 g Sat Fat; 3 g Mono Fat; 42 g Carb; 6 g Fiber; 4 g Sugar; 60 mg Calcium; 2 mg Iron; 53 mg Sodium; 35 mg Cholesterol

YIELD: 4 servings

Loup de Mer au Gingembre et Citron Vert
(SEA BASS WITH GINGER AND LIME)

For the vegetables: Preheat a steamer. Add the greens and cook for 3 to 4 minutes or until desired tenderness. Remove greens and press out excess water. Chop, mix in some lime juice, and season to taste. Set aside for later use.

For the fish: Heat the oil in a nonstick pan over medium heat. Add the fillets and brown. Turn over and cook for 2 minutes. Add a little lime juice, pepper, cover, and reduce heat. Cook the fillets until the flesh starts to flake. Transfer to a serving platter and cover with aluminum foil to keep warm. Add the onions, garlic, ginger, wine, remaining lime juice, honey, and rosemary to the pan. Mix well and bring to a boil. Reduce the sauce to end up with approximately 2/3 cup. Add a little cornstarch mixed with water to thicken. Strain and return to pan. Add the parsley and adjust seasonings. Pour over the fillets and serve immediately with the cooked greens.

The fish and vegetables may be refrigerated separately up to 2 days.

The fish and vegetables may be frozen separately up to 1 month.

FOR THE FISH:
Four 5-ounce sea bass fillets
1 tablespoon olive oil
2 ounces onions, diced (about
    1/2 small onion)
1 teaspoon garlic cloves, minced
1/2 cup Chardonnay wine (or other
    wine with lemon lime flavors)
1/2 cup lime juice
1 tablespoon honey
1 tablespoon fresh ginger, minced
2 tablespoons fresh parsley, minced
1 teaspoon fresh rosemary
Cornstarch with a little water
Salt and pepper to taste

FOR THE VEGETABLES:
2 pounds chard, kale, spinach,
    beet greens, or mustard greens,
    cleaned and pat dry
1 lime
Salt and pepper to taste

Chef's Tip: The amount of cornstarch and water mixture may vary depending on the amount of water rendered by the fish and the reduction process. To obtain the right thickness for a sauce: Dip a spoon in the sauce, turn it over, and make a line across with your finger. Tilt the spoon. If the sauce does not run over the line, it is the perfect thickness. If it does, you need to thicken with a little cornstarch and water mixture. After adding them, you will need to bring the sauce to a boil. Also, if it gets too thick, just add a little liquid to thin out.

Wine Suggestion: Chardonnay (with lemon lime flavors).

SERVING SIZE: One 5-ounce sea bass fillet

PER SERVING: 306 Cal (23% from Fat, 51% from Protein, 26% from Carb); 38 g Protein; 8 g Tot Fat; 1 g Sat Fat; 3 g Mono Fat; 19 g Carb; 5 g Fiber; 8 g Sugar; 150 mg Calcium; 5 mg Iron; 611 mg Sodium; 75 mg Cholesterol

YIELD: 4 servings

Maquereaux à l'Ail
(MACKERELS WITH GARLIC CLOVES)

Preheat the oven to 400 degrees F.

For the fish: Sprinkle pepper and a little salt inside the mackerels. Grease the bottom of a baking pan. Blanch the garlic cloves in boiling water for 3 minutes. Slightly crush them on the bottom of the greased pan. Top them with the mackerels and spread the remaining oil over the fish. Bake for 20 to 25 minutes.

For the vegetables: Preheat a steamer. Add the carrots and cook for 4 minutes. Add the zucchini and continue to cook for 2 to 3 minutes or until desired doneness. Transfer to a serving platter and season to taste.

Serve the mackerels with the vegetables and lemon wedges.

The fish and vegetables may be refrigerated separately up to 2 days.

Not recommended for freezing.

Wine Suggestion: A Loire white or a Sauvignon Blanc from California or Australia.

FOR THE FISH:
Four 5-ounce mackerels
16 garlic cloves, peeled
2 tablespoons olive oil
Salt and pepper to taste

FOR THE VEGETABLES:
1 pound carrots, sliced (about 4 large carrots)
1 pound zucchini, sliced (about 3 large zucchinis)
1 lemon, quartered
Salt and pepper to taste

SERVING SIZE: One 5-ounce mackerel

PER SERVING: 436 Cal (54% from Fat, 27% from Protein, 19% from Carb); 30 g Protein; 27 g Tot Fat; 6 g Sat Fat; 13 g Mono Fat; 21 g Carb; 6 g Fiber; 7 g Sugar; 107 mg Calcium; 3 mg Iron; 220 mg Sodium; 99 mg Cholesterol

YIELD: 4 servings

Maquereaux aux Champignons
(MACKERELS WITH MUSHROOMS)

Preheat the oven to 400 degrees F.

For the fish: Season the inside of the mackerels. Prepare four aluminum foils to fit the mackerels. On each foil place 2 lemon slices, 2 tomato slices, a little garlic, and a few mushroom slices. Add one mackerel and spread over it 1 teaspoon mustard. Sprinkle 1 pinch of herbs de Provence. Top with 2 lemon slices, 2 tomato slices, more mushrooms, and parsley. Close the foil, place in a baking dish, and bake for 20 to 25 minutes.

For the vegetables: Bring to a boil just enough water to cover the beans and add 1 teaspoon salt. Add the green beans and simmer for 10 minutes or until desired doneness. Strain and place in a serving plate. Sprinkle lemon juice and season to taste.

FOR THE FISH:
Four 5-ounce mackerels
4 tomatoes
16 lemon slices (about 2 lemons)
8 ounces white mushrooms, skin removed and sliced (about 8 white mushrooms)
4 teaspoons Dijon mustard
4 pinches herbs de Provence
1 tablespoon garlic cloves, minced
2 tablespoons fresh parsley, minced
Salt and pepper to taste

FOR THE VEGETABLES:
2 pounds green beans, washed and trimmed
1 lemon, juiced
Salt and pepper to taste

Serve the mackerels, their vegetables and juices, with the green beans.

The fish and vegetables may be refrigerated separately up to 2 days.

Not recommended for freezing.

Wine Suggestion: A Loire white or a Sauvignon Blanc from California or Australia. You could also try a Provence rosé or a Bourgogne Pinot Noir.

SERVING SIZE: One 5-ounce mackerel

PER SERVING: 451 Cal (42% from Fat, 30% from Protein, 28% from Carb); 36 g Protein; 22 g Tot Fat; 5 g Sat Fat; 8 g Mono Fat; 34 g Carb; 13 g Fiber; 4 g Sugar; 167 mg Calcium; 6 mg Iron; 422 mg Sodium; 107 mg Cholesterol

YIELD: 4 servings

Morue à la Ratatouille et au Feta
(COD FISH WITH RATATOUILLE AND FETA CHEESE)

Make a small X incision into the tops of the tomatoes. Heat some water over high heat and bring to boil. Blanch the tomatoes for 20 seconds. Remove and place in ice-cold water to stop the cooking process. Peel, seed, and dice the tomatoes.

Heat 1 tablespoon of oil in a deep pan over medium heat. Add the onions and sauté until translucent. Add the zucchini, eggplant, bell peppers, garlic, tomatoes, orange juice, herbs de Provence, bay leaf, and bring to a boil. Reduce heat, cover, and cook for 20 minutes.

Sprinkle the fish with a little pepper. Heat 1 tablespoon oil in a skillet and brown the fish on both sides. Slide the fillets into the ratatouille and continue to cook for 15 minutes. (If the ratatouille is very liquid, leave uncovered; if not, cover.) Remove and place the fillets in a serving platter. Cover with aluminum foil to keep warm. If the ratatouille is still too liquid, reduce uncovered over medium heat until it has the consistency of a sauce. Add the parsley, basil, and adjust seasonings. Transfer to a serving bowl, add the feta cheese, and serve immediately with the fillets.

Four 5-ounce cod fillets
2 tablespoons olive oil
1/2 pound zucchini, diced
    (about 2 medium zucchinis)
1/2 pound eggplant, peeled and
    diced (about 1 medium eggplant)
1/2 pound onions, thinly sliced
    (about 1 large onion)
6 ounces red bell peppers, thinly sliced
    (about 1 large red bell pepper)
6 ounces yellow bell peppers, thinly sliced
    (about 1 large yellow bell pepper)
1 tablespoon garlic cloves, minced
1 pound tomatoes (about 3 large tomatoe
2 ounces orange juice
3 tablespoons fresh parsley, minced
5 fresh basil leaves, minced
1 bay leaf
1/2 teaspoon herbs de Provence
4 ounces feta cheese, diced
Salt and pepper to taste

The fish and vegetables may be refrigerated up to 2 days.

The fish and vegetables may be frozen up to 1 month

Wine Suggestion: Chablis, light Pinot Noir, rosé, German Riesling, Gruener Veltliner, or Zinfandel.

SERVING SIZE: One 5-ounce cod fillet

PER SERVING: 354 Cal (36% from Fat, 36% from Protein, 27% from Carb); 33 g Protein; 15 g Tot Fat; 5 g Sat Fat; 7 g Mono Fat; 25 g Carb; 6 g Fiber; 9 g Sugar; 213 mg Calcium; 2 mg Iron; 416 mg Sodium; 86 mg Cholesterol

YIELD: 4 servings

Papilotte de Saumon au Fenouil
(SALMON AND FENNEL PAPILOTTE)

Preheat the oven to 400 degrees F.

For the fish: Prepare a large aluminum foil packet. Place the salmon in the middle. Sprinkle over a little salt, some pepper, and the herbs de Provence. Top with the onions, carrots, and a few fennel slices (see vegetables). Fold the aluminum foil a bit; add the wine, and fennel seeds. Close and place on a baking dish. Bake for 25 to 30 minutes or until the salmon flesh start to flake.

For the vegetables: Heat the oil in a nonstick pan over high heat. Add the onion and sauté until translucent. Add the fennel, garlic, and sauté for 2 minutes. Pour in the vegetable stock, cover, and cook for 15 to 20 minutes over low heat. Mix in the liquor and the yogurt. Add the cayenne pepper and season to taste.

Place the salmon in a serving platter with its vegetables and juices, and serve immediately with the fennel.

The fish and vegetables may be refrigerated separately up to 2 days. If so, blend in the yogurt only after you reheat.

FOR THE FISH:
1 large salmon fillet (20 ounces)
6 ounces onions, sliced (about
    1 medium onion)
4 ounces carrots, sliced (about
    1 large carrot)
1 teaspoon herbs de Provence
1/4 cup Viognier wine (or
    other wine with orange
    and anise flavors)
1 teaspoon fennel seeds
Salt and pepper to taste

FOR THE VEGETABLES
1 tablespoon olive oil
1 1/2 pounds fennel bulbs,
    trimmed and sliced (about
    2 large fennel bulbs)
6 ounces onions, sliced (about
    1 medium onion)
1 tablespoon garlic cloves, minced
1/4 cup vegetable stock
    (low-sodium)
4 ounces yogurt
1 tablespoon anisette or pastis
Pinch cayenne pepper
Salt and pepper to taste

The fish and vegetables may be frozen separately up to 1 month. If so, blend in the yogurt only after you reheat.

Wine Suggestion: Viognier (with orange and anis flavors).

SERVING SIZE: One 5-ounce salmon fillet

PER SERVING: 440 Cal (42% from Fat, 31% from Protein, 28% from Carb); 33 g Protein; 20 g Tot Fat; 4 g Sat Fat; 8 g Mono Fat; 30 g Carb; 8 g Fiber; 9 g Sugar; 195 mg Calcium; 2 mg Iron; 224 mg Sodium; 85 mg Cholesterol

YIELD: 4 servings

Saumon à l'Orange
(SALMON WITH ORANGE SAUCE)

FOR THE FISH:

Four 5-ounce salmon fillets

1 teaspoon canola oil

1 shallot, thinly sliced

2 oranges

1 teaspoon coriander seeds, crushed

1 1/2 cups fresh orange juice

2 tablespoons Grand Marnier

1 tablespoon orange blossom honey

1 teaspoon dried parsley

Cornstarch with a little water

Salt and pepper to taste

FOR THE VEGETABLES:

2 pounds asparagus, trimmed
      (about 32 asparagus spears)

1/2 orange, juiced

Salt and pepper to taste

Preheat the oven to 400 degrees F.

For the fish: Julienne the oranges' zests and blanch them in boiling water for 2 minutes. Remove and set aside for later use. Remove the white outer part from the oranges. Slice the oranges into approximately 3/8-inch slices.

Grease the bottom of a baking pan. Add the salmon and season to taste. Cover the fillets with a pinch of crushed coriander seeds, half of the zests, shallots, and the orange slices. Warm up 1/4 cup orange juice with the remaining coriander seeds. Pour in the fish pan, cover with aluminum foil, and bake for 20 minutes or until the flesh starts to flake.

Transfer the fish and accompaniment to a serving platter. Cover with aluminum foil to keep warm. Place the cooking liquid in a saucepan. Add the remaining zests, orange juice, and honey. Bring to a boil and reduce to 3/4 cup. Add the Grand Marnier and bring to a boil. Thicken with a little cornstarch mixed with water. Strain and return to the pan. Add parsley and season to taste. Pour the sauce over the fish.

For the vegetables: Preheat a steamer. Add the asparagus and cook for 2 to 3 minutes or until desired tenderness. (Some people like crunchy asparagus, like me; others prefer it more mushy.) Transfer the asparagus to a serving plate, sprinkle with a little orange juice, and season to taste.

Serve the salmon with the asparagus.

The fish and vegetables may be refrigerated separately up to 2 days.

The fish and vegetables may be frozen separately up to 1 month.

Wine Suggestion: A fruity Merlot from Chile or California or a Macon Village white.

SERVING SIZE: One 5-ounce salmon fillet

PER SERVING: 461 Cal (36% from Fat, 31% from Protein, 34% from Carb); 36 g Protein; 19 g Tot Fat; 4 g Sat Fat; 7 g Mono Fat; 39 g Carb; 8 g Fiber; 24 g Sugar; 137 mg Calcium; 3 mg Iron; 125 mg Sodium; 88 mg Cholesterol

YIELD: 4 servings

Saumon à l'Aioli de Basilic
(SALMON WITH BASIL AIOLI)

Preheat the broiler.

For the aioli: All the ingredients must be at room temperature for the emulsion to take. In a food processor, purée the garlic and salt to obtain a smooth paste. Pour in a drop of oil and mix until well incorporated. Continue the same way until most of the oil is incorporated. If you add the oil too quickly, the emulsion will not happen. Before adding the last drop of oil, blend in the basil and add a pinch of pepper.

For the fish: Place the salmon fillets on a greased baking pan. Brush olive oil over the fillets and sprinkle with pepper. Broil 3 to 4 minutes. Turn over, brush with oil, sprinkle with pepper, and continue to broil for 3 to 4 minutes or until the flesh starts to flake. Transfer to a serving platter and salt to taste.

FOR THE AIOLI:
6 to 8 large garlic cloves
1 teaspoon salt
2/3 cup olive oil
2 tablespoons fresh basil, minced
Pinch of pepper

FOR THE FISH:
Four 5-ounce salmon fillets
2 teaspoons olive oil
Salt and pepper to taste

FOR THE VEGETABLES:
12 ounces baby carrots
12 ounces broccoli florets (about 1 large head broccoli florets)
1 lemon, quartered
Salt and pepper to taste

For the vegetables: Preheat a steamer. Add the carrots and cook for 4 minutes. Add the broccoli and continue to cook for 2 minutes. Transfer to a serving plate and season to taste. Decorate with lemon wedges.

Serve the salmon and vegetables with the aioli.

The salmon, aioli, and vegetables may be refrigerated separately up to 2 days.

The salmon and vegetables may be frozen separately up to 1 month.

Wine Suggestion: Alsacian Riesling, Provence rosé, or Burgundy Pinot Noir.

SERVING SIZE: One 5-ounce salmon fillet

PER SERVING: 608 Cal (69% from Fat, 20% from Protein, 11% from Carb); 32 g Protein; 48 g Tot Fat; 7 g Sat Fat; 31 g Mono Fat; 17 g Carb; 7 g Fiber; 5 g Sugar; 120 mg Calcium; 3 mg Iron; 734 mg Sodium; 78 mg Cholesterol

YIELD: 4 servings

Chien de Mer au Vin Rouge Epicé
(DOGFISH WITH SPICY RED WINE SAUCE)

Preheat the oven to 425 degrees F.

For the vegetables: In a bowl, blend the cumin, chili powder, cinnamon, coriander, ginger, and allspice. Place the sweet potatoes and carrots in a baking pan. Add the oil, spices, sprinkle with pepper, and mix well. Bake for 30 minutes or until tender.

For the fish: Sprinkle the fish with pepper. Heat the oil in a nonstick pan over medium heat. Add the fish and brown. Turn over and cook for 3 to 4 minutes or until the fish starts to flake. Transfer the fillets to a plate and cover with aluminum foil to keep warm. Add the shallot, garlic, red wine, and peppercorns to the pan. Bring to boil and reduce by half. Add the brown sauce and reduce to 3/4 cup. Strain the sauce and return to the pan. Add the cayenne pepper, parsley, and season to taste.

FOR THE FISH:

Four 5-ounce dogfish fillets

2 teaspoons canola oil

1 shallot, sliced

2 garlic cloves, minced

1/2 cup red wine Côtes du Rhône (Gigondas)

1 cup brown sauce

6 peppercorns, crushed

Pinch cayenne pepper

1 teaspoon dry parsley

Salt and pepper to taste

FOR THE VEGETABLES:

1 1/4 pounds sweet potatoes, peeled and quartered (about 3 large sweet potatoes)

1 pound carrots, peeled and quartered (about 4 large carrots)

2 tablespoons canola oil

1 teaspoon ground cumin

1 teaspoon chili powder

1 teaspoon ground cinnamon

1 teaspoon coriander

1/2 teaspoon ground ginger

1/2 teaspoon ground allspice

Salt and pepper to taste

Place the fillets on a serving platter and pour the hot sauce over. Serve immediately with the baked vegetables.

The fish and vegetables may be refrigerated separately up to 2 days.

The fish and vegetables may be frozen separately up to 1 month.

Note: If dogfish is not available, substitute salmon.

Gigondas is an appellation for a wine from the Côtes du Rhône region. It is stronger than a regular Côtes du Rhône and more appropriate for this dish. You can find it easily in wine stores.

Brown sauce is a concentrated sauce made out of brown stock (highly concentrated beef stock), mirepoix (onion, carrot, celery), roux (a mixture of flour and butter), tomato purée, and herbs. It is available in most stores in powder form or liquid form. If brown sauce is not available, substitute the 1 cup of brown sauce with 2 cups of beef stock, reduced to 1 cup and thickened with a little cornstarch.

Chef's Secret: Add a little demi-glace (or demiglaze) to emphasize the sauce flavors. Demi-glace is a highly concentrated, rich brown sauce that has been reduced by half. It is easily found in powder and paste form in grocery stores, in specialty stores, or over the Internet. It really adds tremendous flavor to finish a sauce without the fat you would get with butter.

Wine Suggestion: Côtes du Rhône (Gigondas).

SERVING SIZE: One 5-ounce dogfish fillet

PER SERVING: 473 Cal (37% from Fat, 29% from Protein, 34% from Carb); 33 g Protein; 19 g Tot Fat; 2 g Sat Fat; 9 g Mono Fat; 39 g Carb; 8 g Fiber; 11 g Sugar; 124 mg Calcium; 3 mg Iron; 365 mg Sodium; 78 mg Cholesterol

YIELD: 4 servings

Thon Basquais
(TUNA BASQUE STYLE)

Cook the rice according to package instructions.

Make a small X incision on the top and bottom of the tomatoes. Blanch the tomatoes for 20 seconds. Place in ice-cold water to stop the cooking process. Peel, seed, and dice the tomatoes.

Heat 2 teaspoons olive oil in a deep nonstick pan over high heat. Add the onions and sauté until translucent. Add the garlic, bell peppers, thyme, oregano, and sauté for 3 minutes over medium heat. Sprinkle the flour and mix well. Add the tomatoes and continue to cook for 3 to 4 minutes.

Meanwhile, heat the remaining oil in a nonstick skillet over high heat. Add the fish and brown on both sides. Slide the fish into the vegetables, cover, and continue to cook for 15 to 20 minutes over low heat.

Transfer the fish to a serving platter. If necessary, thicken the sauce over medium heat. Add to the fish and serve immediately with the rice.

The fish and rice may be refrigerated separately up to 2 days.

The fish and rice may be frozen separately up to 1 month.

Wine Suggestion: Côtes du Rhône or a red from Navara or Beaujolais. Or try a Graves white.

Four 5-ounce tuna fillets
1 tablespoon olive oil
1 pound onions, sliced (about 2 large onions)
2 pounds tomatoes (about 6 large tomatoes)
8 ounces green bell peppers, ribs and seeds removed, sliced (about 1 large green bell pepper)
1 tablespoon flour
3 garlic cloves, minced
1 pinch dry thyme
1 pinch dry oregano
2 tablespoons fresh parsley, minced
1/2 cup brown rice
Salt and pepper to taste

SERVING SIZE: One 5-ounce tuna fillet

PER SERVING: 443 Cal (26% from Fat, 35% from Protein, 39% from Carb); 39 g Protein; 13 g Tot Fat; 3 g Sat Fat; 6 g Mono Fat; 44 g Carb; 6 g Fiber; 7 g Sugar; 70 mg Calcium; 3 mg Iron; 85 mg Sodium; 54 mg Cholesterol

YIELD: 4 servings

Tian de Sardines
(BAKED SARDINES WITH GREENS)

Four 5-ounce sardines

2 tablespoons olive oil

8 ounces onions, sliced (about 1 large onion)

1 pound Swiss chard

1 pound spinach

3 garlic cloves, minced

1/3 cup milk

1/4 cup fresh parsley, minced

1 teaspoon fresh thyme, minced

2 pinches nutmeg

4 tablespoons Parmesan cheese

1 tablespoon almond meal

Salt and pepper to taste

Preheat the oven to 375 degrees F.

Remove the head, skin, and bones from the sardines (this can be done at the fish market).

Blanch the spinach and Swiss chard for 2 minutes in boiling salted water. Drain and press to remove excess water. Chop the spinach and Swiss chard.

Heat 1 tablespoon olive oil in a nonstick pan over medium heat. Add the onion and sauté until translucent. Add the garlic, spinach, Swiss chard, and cook for 2 minutes, mixing constantly. Mix in the almond meal. Add the milk, 2 tablespoons Parmesan cheese, parsley, thyme, nutmeg, and season to taste.

Pour the mixture in a greased baking dish and slide in the sardines. Sprinkle the remaining Parmesan cheese and drizzle 1 tablespoon olive oil. Cover and bake for 20 to 25 minutes.

The fish and vegetables may be refrigerated separately up to 2 days.

Not recommended for freezing.

Wine Suggestion: Very dry Chardonnay or Assyrtiko from Santorini.

SERVING SIZE: One 5-ounce sardine

PER SERVING: 413 Cal (49% from Fat, 34% from Protein, 17% from Carb); 36 g Protein; 23 g Tot Fat; 6 g Sat Fat; 11 g Mono Fat; 19 g Carb; 7 g Fiber; 6 g Sugar; 434 mg Calcium; 7 mg Iron; 562 mg Sodium; 92 mg Cholesterol

YIELD: 4 servings

Daube de Thon
(TUNA DAUBE)

FOR THE FISH:

Eight 5-ounce tuna fillets

8 small anchovy fillets (canned) drained and pat dry

2 teaspoons olive oil

1 pound onions, diced (about 2 large onions)

8 large tomatoes

6 garlic cloves

1 bouquet garni

2 cups Chardonnay wine (or other citrus and buttery wine)

Salt and pepper to taste

1 cup wild rice

FOR THE MARINADE:

6 ounces olive oil

2 lemons, juiced

Pinch pepper

For the marinade: Mix the oil, lemon juice, and pepper in a bowl.

For the fish: Make two small incisions into each tuna fillet. In each incision, place one anchovy fillet. Place the tuna fillets in a plastic bag. Add the marinade and seal. Mix carefully and refrigerate for at least one hour.

Meanwhile, cook the rice according to package instructions.

Make a small X incision on the top and bottom of the tomatoes. Blanch the tomatoes for 20 seconds. Remove and place in ice-cold water to stop the cooking process. Peel, seed, and dice the tomatoes. Set aside.

Preheat the oven to 350 degrees F. Remove the fish from the bag and pat dry with paper towels. Heat 2 teaspoons of olive oil in a nonstick pan over high heat. Add the tuna and brown on both sides over high heat. Transfer the fish to a plate.

Deglaze the pan with a little water. To deglaze, add a liquid (such as wine, stock, or water) and swirl to dissolve cooked particles on the bottom or side of the pan.

Add the onions and slightly brown. Add the tomatoes, garlic, bouquet garni, white wine, and bring to a boil.

Transfer half of the vegetables to a greased casserole. Add the fish and top with the remaining vegetables and wine. Cover and bake for 20 to 25 minutes.

Remove the fish and place on a serving platter. Cover with aluminum foil to keep warm. Remove the bouquet garni. Thicken the sauce by simmering over medium heat. Adjust seasonings and pour over the tuna fillets. Serve immediately with the wild rice.

This dish may be refrigerated for 2 days.

This dish may be frozen up to 1 month.

Wine Suggestion: Chardonnay (citrus and buttery).

SERVING SIZE: One 5-ounce tuna fillet

PER SERVING: 454 Cal (28% from Fat, 39% from Protein, 33% from Carb); 41 g Protein; 13 g Tot Fat; 3 g Sat Fat; 5 g Mono Fat; 35 g Carb; 4 g Fiber; 3 g Sugar; 93 mg Calcium; 3 mg Iron; 535 mg Sodium; 65 mg Cholesterol

YIELD: 8 servings

Daurade au Safran
(SEA BREAM WITH SAFFRON)

FOR THE FISH:

Four 6-ounce sea bream fillets

2 teaspoons olive oil

1 teaspoon garlic cloves, minced

3 to 4 saffron sprigs

1/2 cup Chardonnay wine
(or other citrus and buttery wine)

1/2 cup fish or vegetable stock or
combination (low-sodium)

1 large tomato, peeled, seeded, and diced

2 tablespoons fresh salad herbs, minced

Pinch paprika

1/2 lemon

Cornstarch with a little water

Salt and pepper to taste

For the fish: Make a small X incision on the top and bottom of the tomatoes. Blanch the tomatoes for 20 seconds. Place in ice-cold water to stop the cooking process. Peel, seed, and dice the tomatoes.

Heat the oil in a nonstick pan over medium heat. Add the fillets and brown. Turn over carefully and sauté for 1 minute. Sprinkle a little pepper, lemon juice, and continue to cook over medium heat until the fillets are done. Remove the fillets and set aside on a serving platter. Cover with aluminum foil to keep warm.

Add the garlic, saffron, wine, and paprika to the lemon juice mixture still in the pan. Bring to a boil until it is reduced by half to concentrate the flavors. Add the stock and any juices rendered by the fillets (that is, any liquid on the plate with the fillets), and bring to a boil. Strain the sauce and return to pan. Thicken with a little cornstarch mixed with water. Add the tomatoes, herbs, and bring to a boil. Pour over the fillets and serve immediately.

For the vegetables: Heat the oil in a nonstick pan over high heat. Add the leeks and sauté until translucent. Add the bell peppers, carrots, and garlic. Cook for 3 to 4 minutes over medium heat. Add a little lemon juice, herbs, and season to taste. Serve immediately with the fish.

The fish and vegetables may be refrigerated separately up to 2 days.

Chef's Tip: The amount of cornstarch and water mixture may vary depending on the amount of water rendered by the fish and the reduction process. To obtain the right thickness for a sauce: Dip a spoon in the sauce, turn it over, and make a line across with your finger. Tilt the spoon. If the sauce does not run over the line, it is the perfect thickness. If it does, you need to thicken with a little cornstarch and water mixture. After adding them, you will need to bring the sauce to a boil. Also, if it gets too thick, just add a little liquid to thin out.

FOR THE VEGETABLES:

1 teaspoon olive oil

1 teaspoon garlic cloves, minced

8 ounces leeks, julienned (about 1 large leek)

8 ounces green bell peppers, julienned (about 1 large bell pepper)

8 ounces red bell peppers, julienned (about 1 large red bell pepper)

8 ounces carrots, julienned (about 2 large carrots)

2 tablespoons fresh salad herbs, minced

1/2 lemon

Salt and pepper to taste

Chef's Secret: If a fishy sauce is not your favorite, use vegetable stock. My favorite is to use half fish and half vegetable stock.

Wine Suggestion: Chardonnay (citrus and buttery).

SERVING SIZE: One 6-ounce sea bream fillet

PER SERVING: 366 Cal (22% from Fat, 50% from Protein, 28% from Carb); 44 g Protein; 9 g Tot Fat; 2 g Sat Fat; 4 g Mono Fat; 24 g Carb; 5 g Fiber; 9 g Sugar; 107 mg Calcium; 3 mg Iron; 305 mg Sodium; 90 mg Cholesterol

YIELD: 4 servings

Rascasse au Coulis de Poivron
(OCEAN PERCH WITH BELL PEPPER COULIS)

FOR THE FISH:
Four 5-ounce ocean perch fillets
2 tablespoons olive oil
1 pound red bell peppers (about
   3 large red bell peppers)
1 shallot, minced
1 teaspoon garlic cloves, minced
1 teaspoon lemon juice
1 tablespoon fresh basil, chopped
Salt and pepper to taste

FOR THE VEGETABLES:
2 pounds eggplants, sliced medium
   (about 3 large eggplants)
2 tablespoons olive oil
Salt and pepper to taste

Preheat the broiler.

For the fish: Place the red bell peppers on a baking sheet and char on all sides. If you have a gas stovetop, you may char the bell peppers over the flames. Once blackened on all sides, place in a paper bag and seal. Let stand for 10 minutes. Peel and seed the bell peppers. Remove ribs and quarter. Purée in a blender with the shallot, garlic, 1 tablespoon olive oil, basil, and lemon juice. Thin out with a little water and season to taste.

Heat 1 tablespoon olive oil in a nonstick pan over medium heat. Add the fillets and brown. Turn over and continue to cook for 2 minutes. Add a little coulis, cover, reduce heat, and continue to cook until the flesh starts to flake. Transfer the fillets to a serving platter. Cover with aluminum foil to keep warm. Add the remaining coulis and bring to boil over medium heat. Adjust seasonings and pour over the fillets.

For the vegetables: Brush the eggplant slices with olive oil, season to taste, and brown under the broiler on both sides. Time will vary depending on the thickness, so it is best to keep a close eye on the eggplant. Remove and place on a serving platter.

Serve the fillets with the eggplants.

The fish and vegetables may be refrigerated separately up to 2 days.

The fish may be frozen up to 1 month. Not recommended for the eggplant.

Wine Suggestion: Alsacian Riesling or Montrachet or Côtes de Provence (white or red).

SERVING SIZE: One 5-ounce ocean perch fillet

PER SERVING: 335 Cal (41% from Fat, 36% from Protein, 24% from Carb); 31 g Protein; 16 g Tot Fat; 2 g Sat Fat; 10 g Mono Fat; 20 g Carb; 10 g Fiber; 10 g Sugar; 145 mg Calcium; 2 mg Iron; 95 mg Sodium; 128 mg Cholesterol

YIELD: 4 servings

Red Snapper with Basil and Oregano

Preheat the oven to 400 degrees F. Grease a baking pan.

Make a small X incision into the tops and the bottoms of the tomatoes. Heat some water over high heat and bring to boil. Blanch the tomatoes for 20 seconds. Remove and place in ice-cold water to stop the cooking process. Peel, seed, and dice the tomatoes.

Cook the rice according to package directions.

Sprinkle a little pepper over the fillets. Heat 2 teaspoons of oil in a nonstick pan (ovenproof) over medium heat. Add the fish and brown on both sides. Remove the fish and set aside, covered.

Four 5-ounce red snapper fillets
1 tablespoon olive oil
6 ounces onions, diced (about 1 medium onion)
1 tablespoon garlic cloves, minced
1 1/2 pound tomatoes (about 4 large tomatoes)
12 ounces artichoke hearts, chopped (about 1 1/2 cup)
2 tablespoons fresh basil, chopped
2 teaspoons fresh oregano, chopped
1 teaspoon fresh thyme, chopped
2 tablespoons fresh parsley, chopped
1/2 cup brown rice
Salt and pepper to taste

Deglaze the pan with water. To deglaze, add water and swirl to dissolve cooked particles on the bottom or side of the pan. Discard the water. Heat the remaining oil over high heat. Add the onions, and sauté until translucent. Stir in the garlic, tomatoes, and herbs. Bring to a boil and reduce for 5 minutes over medium heat. Mix in the artichokes and season to taste. Pour half the vegetables in the bottom of the baking pan, add the fillets, and top with the remaining vegetables. Cover and bake for 15 to 20 minutes. Serve immediately with the rice.

The fish and rice may be refrigerated separately up to 2 days.

The fish and rice may be frozen separately up to 1 month.

Wine Suggestion: Sauvignon Blanc or a light Pinot Noir or Provence rosé.

SERVING SIZE: One 5-ounce red snapper fillet

PER SERVING: 394 Cal (17% from Fat, 44% from Protein, 39% from Carb); 44 g Protein; 8 g Tot Fat; 1 g Sat Fat; 3 g Mono Fat; 39 g Carb; 7 g Fiber; 3 g Sugar; 112 mg Calcium; 3 mg Iron; 146 mg Sodium; 67 mg Cholesterol

YIELD: 4 servings

Sardines à l'Escabèche
(SARDINES ESCABÈCHE STYLE)

FOR THE FISH:

Four 5-ounce sardines

2 tablespoons olive oil

4 ounces onions, diced small (about 1 small onion)

2 ounces carrots, diced small (about 1 small carrot)

2 ounces celery, diced small (about 1 large celery stalk)

1 leek (white part only), diced small

1 tablespoon garlic cloves, minced

1 bouquet garni

1 lemon, zest plus juice

1 cup white wine (lemony Chardonnay or Sauvignon Blanc)

4 tablespoons Xères or sherry vinegar

2 pinches paprika

1/2 cup fish or vegetable stock or a combination (low-sodium)

Salt and pepper to taste

For the fish: Remove the head and bones from the sardines (this can be done at the fish market).

Heat 1 tablespoon of oil in a nonstick pan over medium heat. Add the sardines and cook for 3 minutes or until cooked through. Do not turn over because they are very fragile. Remove and place the sardines in a serving platter. Cover with aluminum foil to keep warm. Deglaze the pan with water. To deglaze, add water and swirl to dissolve cooked particles on the bottom or side of the pan. Discard the water.

Heat the remaining oil in the pan over high heat. Add the onions, leek, and cook for 2 minutes. Add the carrots, celery, garlic, wine, lemon zest, lemon juice, vinegar, bouquet garni, paprika, and cook for 10 minutes over medium heat. Add the stock and reduce by half. Adjust seasonings, remove bouquet garni, and spread over the sardines. Cover to keep warm.

For the vegetables: Heat the oil in a sauté pan over medium heat. Cook the pearl onions until golden brown. Add the garlic, lima beans, herbs de Provence, and season to taste. Add 1/4 cup stock, mix well, and bring to a boil. Continue to cook until the stock is almost evaporated. Taste and adjust seasonings.

Serve the sardines with the vegetables and lemon wedges.

This dish may be refrigerated up to 2 days.

Not recommended for freezing.

Chef's Secret: If a fishy sauce is not your favorite, use vegetable stock. My favorite is to use half fish and half vegetable stock.

Wine Suggestion: Chardonnay (lemony) or Sauvignon Blanc.

FOR THE VEGETABLES:

1 tablespoon olive oil

1 pound pearl onions, peeled

1 cup frozen baby lima beans

1 teaspoon garlic cloves, minced

1 pinch herbs de Provence

1 lemon, quartered

1/4 cup vegetable stock (low-sodium)

Salt and pepper to taste

SERVING SIZE: One 5-ounce sardine

PER SERVING: 473 Cal (48% from Fat, 26% from Protein, 26% from Carb); 29 g Protein; 24 g Tot Fat; 4 g Sat Fat; 13 g Mono Fat; 29 g Carb; 5 g Fiber; 11 g Sugar; 178 mg Calcium; 3 mg Iron; 261 mg Sodium; 85 mg Cholesterol

YIELD: 4 servings

Espadon aux Noix
(SWORDFISH WITH WALNUTS)

FOR THE FISH:
Four 5-ounce swordfish steaks
2 teaspoons canola oil
1/2 lemon, juiced
2 ounces walnuts (about 1/2 cup walnuts)
1 slice white bread
4 tablespoons milk
2 teaspoons garlic cloves, minced
3/4 ounce olive oil
Pinch nutmeg
Salt and pepper to taste

FOR THE VEGETABLES:
1 pound yellow squash, chopped
    (about 3 large yellow squash)
1 pound tomatoes, quartered and seeded
    (about 3 large tomatoes)
1 teaspoon olive oil
1 teaspoon garlic cloves, minced
1/2 lemon, juiced
2 pinches dried Italian herbs
Salt and pepper to taste

Preheat the oven to 425 degrees F.

For the vegetables: In a casserole, blend the squash, tomatoes, oil, garlic, lemon juice, Italian herbs, and season to taste. Bake for 20 to 25 minutes, mixing halfway through the cooking time.

For the fish: Soak the bread in 1 1/2 tablespoon milk. In a blender, purée the walnuts, garlic, 3/4 ounce olive oil, and nutmeg. Add the bread and mix well. Blend in 1 1/2 tablespoon milk and season to taste.

Heat the oil in a nonstick pan over high heat. Add the fish and brown. Turn over and sauté for 2 minutes. Sprinkle pepper over the fish. Add the lemon juice, cover, reduce heat, and continue to cook for another 3 to 4 minutes or until the flesh starts to flake.

Warm up 1 tablespoon milk and mix in the walnut paste. Serve immediately with the fish and vegetables.

The fish and vegetables may be refrigerated separately up to 2 days.

The fish and vegetables may be frozen separately up to 1 month.

This walnut paste can be used as a dip for vegetables, for croutons, sandwich base, salad dressing base, and so on.

Wine Suggestion: Italian Pinot Grigio, Sancerre, or Pouilly Fumé.

SERVING SIZE: One 5-ounce swordfish steak

PER SERVING: 414 Cal (52% from Fat, 32% from Protein, 17% from Carb); 34 g Protein; 25 g Tot Fat; 4 g Sat Fat; 10 g Mono Fat; 18 g Carb; 5 g Fiber; 4 g Sugar; 88 mg Calcium; 3 mg Iron; 184 mg Sodium; 57 mg Cholesterol

YIELD: 4 servings

THE Saint Tropez Diet

Meat Entrees

Côtes d'Agneau Persillées
(LAMB CHOPS WITH HERBS)

Preheat the oven to 400 degrees F.

In a bowl, combine the garlic, parsley, bread crumbs, herbs de Provence, a pinch of salt, and a pinch of pepper. Add the mustard and just enough oil to bind.

Heat 1 teaspoon olive oil in a nonstick pan over high heat. Add the lamb chops and quickly brown on both sides. Remove from heat. Place the chops on a greased baking pan. Spread the bread crumbs mixture over the chops and press hard. Bake for 10 minutes for medium rare or up to 15 minutes for well-done.

This dish goes well with Couscous with Vegetables (see page 262).

The lamb and couscous may be refrigerated separately up to 5 days.

The lamb and couscous may be frozen separately up to 1 month.

Wine Suggestion: Break out your best red. Try a Bordeaux or Côtes du Rhône, or even the best Cabernet from California or Chile that you have in your possession.

Eight 3 1/2-ounce loin lamb chops (about 1 3/4 pounds total)
2 tablespoons olive oil
2 tablespoons garlic cloves, minced
1 tablespoon parsley, minced
4 tablespoons bread crumbs
1 tablespoon herbs de Provence, minced
3 tablespoons Dijon mustard
Salt and pepper to taste

SERVING SIZE: Two 3 1/2-ounce loin lamb chops

PER SERVING: 363 Cal (44% from Fat, 48% from Protein, 8% from Carb); 42 g Protein; 17 g Tot Fat; 5 g Sat Fat; 9 g Mono Fat; 7 g Carb; 1 g Fiber; 1 g Sugar; 51 mg Calcium; 5 mg Iron; 309 mg Sodium; 127 mg Cholesterol (lamb)

YIELD: 4 servings

Daube Provençal
(BEEF STEW PROVENCE STYLE)

3 pounds beef (stew meat)

4 ounces Canadian bacon, diced

1 pounds onions, diced (about 2 large onions)

12 ounces carrots, sliced (about 3 large carrots)

5 garlic cloves, minced

1 bottle red wine such as Côtes du Rhône (Grenache), Australian Shiraz, Bordeaux Merlot

6 peppercorns

1/2 orange, zest plus juice

2 parsley branches

1 bouquet garni

1 cup tomatoes

3 tablespoons pitted black olives

2 pounds potatoes (about 4 medium potatoes)

Salt and pepper to taste

In a large bowl place the meat, bacon, onions, carrots, garlic, wine, peppercorn, orange zest, orange juice, and parsley branches. Marinade overnight in the refrigerator.

Make a small X incision on the top and bottom of the tomatoes. Blanch the tomatoes for 20 seconds. Place in ice-cold water to stop the cooking process. Peel, seed, and dice the tomatoes.

Preheat the oven to 325 degrees F. Grease a Dutch oven. Add the meat, marinade ingredients, bouquet garni, tomatoes, and olives. Cover and cook for 2 1/2 to 3 hours.

Half an hour before the meat is done, immerse the potatoes in cold water and add 1 teaspoon of salt. Bring to boil and cook until tender. Strain and serve with the daube.

Before serving the daube, remove any fat floating on the surface with a spoon. This process will decrease the fat content and therefore reduce the final calorie count.

The daube and potatoes may be refrigerated separately up to 5 days.

The daube may be frozen separately up to 1 month.

If a Dutch oven is not available, use an ovenproof stew pot that is wide rather than tall.

Wine Suggestion: Côtes du Rhône (Grenache), Australian Shiraz, Bordeaux Merlot, or a California Cabernet.

SERVING SIZE: 4 ounces beef. This is an estimate. It is hard to tell since it may vary based on the cooking, water content, and fat content released during the cooking time.

PER SERVING: 600 Cal (50% from Fat, 25% from Protein, 25% from Carb); 37 g Protein; 33 g Tot Fat; 13 g Sat Fat; 14 g Mono Fat; 36 g Carb; 5 g Fiber; 6 g Sugar; 60 mg Calcium; 5 mg Iron; 310 mg Sodium; 123 mg Cholesterol

YIELD: 8 servings

Poitrine de Canard aux Baies
(DUCK BREAST WITH BERRIES)

Preheat the oven to 350 degrees F.

Cook the rice according to package instructions.

Score the duck breast fat with diagonal cuts from one end to the other, and repeat from the other side. This will create a diamond shape in the fat. Do not cut through the meat. Sprinkle some pepper on the flesh side.

Heat the oil in an ovenproof sauté pan over high heat. Add the duck breasts on the fat side and sauté until golden brown, approximately 3 minutes. Turn over and continue to cook for 2 minutes. Place in the oven for 5 minutes (rare) to 10 minutes (well-done). Remove the breasts from the pan and set aside in a serving platter. Cover with aluminum foil to keep warm.

Four 6-ounce duck breasts
1 teaspoon canola oil
1 shallot, sliced
2 tablespoons pomegranate
    or raspberry vinegar
1/2 cup Zinfandel or Syrah
    (or other wine with
    berry flavors)
1 cup chicken stock (low-fat
    and low-sodium)
8 ounces blueberries
1 fresh thyme branch
1 fresh rosemary branch
2 juniper berries
Cornstarch and a little water
1/2 cup wild rice
Salt and pepper to taste

Discard excess fat from the pan. Add the shallot, vinegar, wine, and boil until reduced by half. Add the stock, half the blueberries, thyme, rosemary, juniper berries, and boil until reduced by half. Pass through a sieve, pressing hard to extract all the juices, and return the liquid to the pan. Add any juices rendered by the duck and bring to a boil. Reduce a little more and thicken with a little cornstarch mixed with water. Adjust seasonings and add the remaining blueberries. Bring to a boil and pour over the duck breasts. Serve immediately with the wild rice.

The duck and rice may be refrigerated separately up to 5 days.

Freezing is not recommended.

Note: 25 percent or more of fat will be discarded during the cooking process. The amount of fat may vary depending on the type of breast you get, so the final calorie count may also vary.

Chef's Tip: The amount of cornstarch and water mixture may vary depending on the amount of water rendered by the duck and the reduction process. To obtain the right thickness for a sauce: Dip a spoon in the sauce, turn it over, and make a line across with your finger. Tilt the spoon. If the sauce does not run over the line, it is the perfect thickness. If it does, you need to thicken with a little cornstarch and water mixture. After adding them, you will need to bring the sauce to a boil. Also, if it gets too thick, just add a little liquid to thin out.

Chef's Secret: Add a little demi-glace (or demiglaze) to emphasize the sauce flavors. Demi-glace is a highly concentrated rich brown sauce that has been reduced by half. It is easily found in powder or paste form in grocery stores, in specialty stores, or over the Internet. It really adds tremendous flavor to finish a sauce without the fat you would get with butter.

Wine Suggestion: Zinfandel or Syrah (berry flavors).

SERVING SIZE: One 6-ounce duck breast

PER SERVING: 570 Cal (27% from Fat, 30% from Protein, 43% from Carb); 41 g Protein; 16 g Tot Fat; 4 g Sat Fat; 7 g Mono Fat; 59 g Carb; 4 g Fiber; 1 g Sugar; 51 mg Calcium; 9 mg Iron; 869 mg Sodium; 132 mg Cholesterol

YIELD: 4 servings

Filet de Porc au Coulis de Tomates
(PORK LOIN WITH TOMATO COULIS)

Make a small X incision on the top and bottom of the tomatoes. Blanch the tomatoes for 20 seconds. Place in ice-cold water to stop the cooking process. Peel, seed, and dice the tomatoes.

Sprinkle the pork loins with pepper. Heat the oil in a deep pan over high heat. Add the loins and brown on both sides. Add the garlic, shallots, tomatoes, sugar, and reduce heat to medium. Sprinkle the flour over the vegetables and mix well. Continue to cook for 2 minutes. Add the wine, stock, tomato paste, rosemary, and bring to a boil. Cover and cook for 25 minutes over low heat.

Remove loins and set aside in a serving platter. Cover with aluminum foil to keep warm. Remove the rosemary and purée the sauce with a hand mixer or in a blender. Return to the pan and reduce the sauce to concentrate its flavors. If necessary, thicken with a little cornstarch mixed with water. Add the basil, parsley, any rendered pork juices, and bring to a boil. Adjust seasonings and pour over the loins.

Four 5-ounce pork loins
1 tablespoon olive oil
3 garlic cloves, minced
2 shallots, minced
2 pounds tomatoes (about
    6 large tomatoes)
Pinch sugar
1 tablespoon flour
1/2 cup Chardonnay wine
    (or other lemony and
    buttery wine)
1/2 cup veal stock
    (low-fat and low-sodium)
1 teaspoon tomato paste
1 fresh rosemary branch
2 tablespoons fresh basil, minced
2 tablespoons fresh
    parsley, minced
Cornstarch and water
Salt and pepper to taste

This dish goes well with Risotto with Olives (see page 279).

The pork and risotto may be refrigerated separately up to 5 days.

The pork and risotto may be frozen separately up to 1 month.

Chef's Tip: The amount of cornstarch and water mixture may vary depending on the amount of water rendered by the pork and the reduction process. To obtain the right thickness for a sauce: Dip a spoon in the sauce, turn it over, and make a line across with your finger. Tilt the spoon. If the sauce does not run over the line, it is the perfect thickness. If it does, you need to thicken with a little cornstarch and water mixture. After adding them, you will need to bring the sauce to a boil. Also, if it gets too thick, just add a little liquid to thin out.

Wine Suggestion: Chardonnay (lemony and buttery).

SERVING SIZE: One 5-ounce pork loin

PER SERVING: 333 Cal (39% from Fat, 42% from Protein, 19% from Carb); 33 g Protein; 14 g Tot Fat; 4 g Sat Fat; 7 g Mono Fat; 15 g Carb; 3 g Fiber; 2 g Sugar; 48 mg Calcium; 2 mg Iron; 304 mg Sodium; 81 mg Cholesterol (pork)

YIELD: 4 servings

Poitrine de Poulet aux Champignons Sauvages
(CHICKEN BREAST WITH WILD MUSHROOMS)

For the chicken: Heat the oil in a nonstick pan over high heat. Add the chicken and brown on both sides. Add the shallots, garlic, wine, and reduce by half. Add half of the chicken stock, 1 sprig of rosemary, and bring to a boil. Reduce heat, cover, and simmer for 10 to 15 minutes or until the chicken is cooked through.

Transfer the chicken breasts to a serving platter. Cover with aluminum foil to keep warm. Add the remaining stock and reduce to a little less than 1 cup. Thicken with a little cornstarch and water. Add the parsley, any rendered chicken juices, and bring to a boil. Adjust seasonings and pour over the chicken.

For the mushrooms: Heat oil in a nonstick pan over medium heat. Add the mushrooms and cook until almost cooked through. Add the chestnuts, mix well, season to taste, and continue to cook for 2 to 3 minutes. Add a little sauce from the chicken and mix well.

Serve the chicken breasts with the mushrooms and chestnuts.

FOR THE CHICKEN:
Four 5-ounce skinless
   chicken breasts
2 teaspoons olive oil
2 shallots, minced
3 garlic cloves, minced
1/2 cup red wine (earthy
   Syrah, Shiraz, or
   Barbaresco)
1 cup chicken stock (low-
   fat and low-sodium)
2 sprigs fresh rosemary
1 tablespoon fresh
   parsley, minced
Cornstarch plus water
Salt and pepper to taste

FOR THE MUSHROOMS:
2 teaspoons olive oil
1 pound wild mushrooms,
   cleaned and sliced
1 pound cooked chestnuts
Salt and pepper to taste

The chicken and vegetables may be refrigerated separately up to 5 days.

Not recommended for freezing.

Chef's Tip: The amount of cornstarch and water mixture may vary depending on the amount of water rendered by the chicken and the reduction process. To obtain the right thickness for a sauce: Dip a spoon in the sauce, turn it over, and make a line across with your finger. Tilt the spoon. If the sauce does not run over the line, it is the perfect thickness. If it does, you need to thicken with a little cornstarch and water mixture. After adding them, you will need to bring the sauce to a boil. Also, if it gets too thick, just add a little liquid to thin out.

Chef's Secret: Add a little demi-glace (or demiglaze) to emphasize the sauce flavors. Demi-glace is a highly concentrated rich brown sauce that has been reduced by half. It is easily found in powder or paste form in grocery stores, in specialty stores, or over the Internet. It really adds tremendous flavor to finish a sauce without the fat you would get with butter.

Wine Suggestion: Earthy Syrah, Shiraz, or Barbaresco.

SERVING SIZE: One 5-ounce skinless chicken breast

PER SERVING: 441 Cal (21% from Fat, 32% from Protein, 47% from Carb); 34 g Protein; 10 g Tot Fat; 2 g Sat Fat; 5 g Mono Fat; 50 g Carb; 3 g Fiber; 5 g Sugar; 87 mg Calcium; 5 mg Iron; 284 mg Sodium; 92 mg Cholesterol

YIELD: 4 servings

Poitrine de Poulet à l'Ail
(Chicken Breast with Garlic Cloves)

FOR THE CHICKEN:
Four 5-ounce skinless
  chicken breasts
2 teaspoons canola oil
1 1/4 cups garlic cloves,
  peeled
1/4 cup Chardonnay wine
  (lemon and herbs)
1 cup chicken stock (low-
  fat and low-sodium)
1/2 lemon, juiced
1 sprig fresh thyme
1 sprig fresh rosemary
1 bay leaf
Cornstarch plus water
Salt and pepper to taste

Preheat the oven to 425 degrees F.

For the vegetables: Place the potatoes and carrots in a baking pan. Mix in 2 teaspoons oil and sprinkle with paprika. Bake for 25 minutes. Add the red onions, red bell peppers, broccoli, garlic, minced herbs, a little more oil, sprinkle with pepper, and mix well. Continue to bake for 15 to 20 minutes. Sprinkle with salt before serving.

For the chicken: Heat the oil in a nonstick pan over high heat. Add the chicken breasts and brown on both sides. Transfer the chicken breasts to a plate.

Deglaze the pan with a little water and add the garlic cloves. To deglaze, add a liquid (such as wine, stock, or water) and swirl to dissolve cooked particles on the bottom or side of the pan. Sauté until the cloves are slightly brown. Add the chicken, wine, 1/2 cup stock, lemon juice, thyme sprig, rosemary sprig, and bay leaf. Bring to boil, cover, reduce heat, and cook for 15 to 20 minutes or until the chicken is cooked through. Place the chicken breasts and garlic cloves in a serving platter. Cover with aluminum foil to keep warm.

Add the remaining stock and boil until reduced to end up with 3/4 cup. Strain and return to the pan. Thicken with a little cornstarch and water mixture. Add any rendered chicken juices, bring to a boil, and adjust seasonings. Pour over the chicken breasts.

Serve the chicken with the baked vegetables.

The chicken and vegetables may be refrigerated separately up to 5 days.

The chicken and vegetables may be frozen separately up to 1 month.

Chef's Tip: The amount of cornstarch and water mixture may vary depending on the amount of water rendered by the chicken and the reduction process. To obtain the right thickness for a sauce: Dip a spoon in the sauce, turn it over, and make a line across with your finger. Tilt the spoon. If the sauce does not run over the line, it is the perfect thickness. If it does, you need to thicken with a little cornstarch and water mixture. After adding them, you will need to bring the sauce to a boil. Also, if it gets too thick, just add a little liquid to thin out.

Chef's Secret: Add a little demi-glace (or demiglaze) to emphasize the sauce flavors. Demi-glace is a highly concentrated rich brown sauce that has been reduced by half. It is easily found in powder or paste form in grocery stores, in specialty stores, or over the Internet. It really adds tremendous flavor to finish a sauce without the fat you would get with butter.

Wine Suggestion: Chardonnay (with lemon and herb flavors).

FOR THE VEGETABLES:

1 tablespoon canola oil

1 pound white potatoes, washed, pat dry, and quartered (about 3 medium white potatoes)

6 ounces carrots, chopped (about 2 medium carrots)

12 ounces broccoli florets (about 1 large head broccoli florets)

6 ounces red onions, quartered (about 1 medium red onion)

6 ounces red bell peppers, chopped (about 1 large red bell pepper)

3 garlic cloves, minced

1 sprig fresh thyme, minced

1 sprig fresh rosemary, minced

1 bay leaf, minced

Salt, pepper, and paprika to taste

SERVING SIZE: One 5-ounce skinless chicken breast

PER SERVING: 497 Cal (20% from Fat, 41% from Protein, 40% from Carb); 50 g Protein; 11 g Tot Fat; 2 g Sat Fat; 5 g Mono Fat; 49 g Carb; 7 g Fiber; 7 g Sugar; 185 mg Calcium; 4 mg Iron; 298 mg Sodium; 109 mg Cholesterol

YIELD: 4 servings

Paupiette de Dinde à l'Italienne
(STUFFED TURKEY BREAST ITALIAN STYLE)

Preheat the oven to 350 degrees F.

For the turkey: Place the turkey breasts between two plastic wrap sheets. Flatten with a mallet until fairly thin. Sprinkle pepper and a pinch of Italian herbs on each breast. Add one slice of ham, one slice of cheese, 2 basil leaves, and roll tightly. Secure with a few toothpicks so it does not unroll.

Heat the oil in a sauté pan over high heat. Add the turkey rolls, placing the folded side down first. Brown and turn over. Once browned, add the shallot, Madeira wine, and half of the chicken stock. Bring to a boil and place in the oven for 10 to 12 minutes. Transfer the rolls on a serving platter and cover with aluminum foil to keep warm. Add the remaining stock and reduce the sauce to end up with less than 1 cup. Thicken with a little cornstarch mixed with water. Add the parsley, any rendered turkey juices, and bring to a boil. Adjust seasonings and pour over the turkey.

Four 4-ounce skinless turkey breasts
1 tablespoon olive oil
4 slices Prosciutto ham
2 ounces goat cheese, sliced in 4 pieces
1 large shallot, thinly sliced
1/4 cup Madeira wine
1 cup chicken stock (low-fat and low-sodium)
4 pinches dried Italian herbs
8 fresh large basil leaves
2 tablespoons fresh parsley, minced
Cornstarch plus a little water
Salt and pepper to taste

This dish goes well with Green Beans with Tomatoes (see page 264).

The turkey and vegetables may be refrigerated separately up to 5 days.

The turkey and vegetables may be frozen separately up to 1 month.

Chef's Tip: The amount of cornstarch and water mixture may vary depending on the amount of water rendered by the turkey and the reduction process. To obtain the right thickness for a sauce: Dip a spoon in the sauce, turn it over, and make a line across with your finger. Tilt the spoon. If the sauce does not run over the line, it is the perfect thickness. If it does, you need to thicken with a little cornstarch and water mixture. After adding them, you will need to bring the sauce to a boil. Also, if it gets too thick, just add a little liquid to thin out.

Chef's Secret: Add a little demi-glace (or demiglaze) to emphasize the sauce flavors. Demi-glace is a highly concentrated rich brown sauce that has been reduced by half. It is easily found in powder or paste form in grocery stores, in specialty stores, or over the Internet. It really adds tremendous flavor to finish a sauce without the fat you would get with butter.

Wine Suggestion: Madeira.

SERVING SIZE: 4-ounce skinless turkey breast

PER SERVING: 326 Cal (46% from Fat, 52% from Protein, 2% from Carb); 40 g Protein; 16 g Tot Fat; 5 g Sat Fat; 7 g Mono Fat; 2 g Carb; 0 g Fiber; 0 g Sugar; 56 mg Calcium; 2 mg Iron; 648 mg Sodium; 100 mg Cholesterol (turkey)

YIELD: 4 servings

Rôti de Porc aux Figues
(Pork Roast with Figs)

Preheat the oven to 350 degrees F.

For the figs: Make an X incision into the top of the figs. Place the figs and the acorn squash (cut side down) into a baking pan. Bring to a boil the orange juice, wine, and honey in a saucepan over high heat. Mix well and pour over the figs and acorn squash. Bake for 30 minutes at 350 degrees F, spooning the sauce over every 10 minutes.

Preheat the broiler. Cover a baking sheet with parchment paper. Spread over the almonds and brown under the broiler. Remove from the pan and set aside for later use.

For the pork: Preheat the oven to 350 degrees F. Place the roast in a roasting pan, rub with a little oil, and sprinkle with pepper. Bake for 1 hour or until the inside temperature reaches 185 degrees F.

Remove the roast from the pan, set aside on a plate, and sprinkle with salt to taste. Cover with aluminum foil to keep warm. Allow 10 to 15 minutes before slicing.

FOR THE MEAT:

20 ounces center loin pork roast (boneless)

1 teaspoon olive oil

1 cup veal stock (low-fat and low-sodium)

1 fresh rosemary branch

3 tablespoons fresh parsley, minced

Salt and pepper to taste

FOR THE FIGS:

2 tablespoons sliced almonds

8 figs

2 acorn squash, halved and seeded

1 orange, juiced

1/2 cup Chardonnay wine (or other wine with vanilla, orange rind, and honey flavor)

2 tablespoons honey

Cornstarch with a little water

Salt and pepper to taste

Deglaze the pan with the stock. To deglaze, add a liquid (such as wine, stock, or water) and swirl to dissolve cooked particles on the bottom or side of the pan. Scrape out all the particles on the bottom of the pan. Transfer to a saucepan and bring to a boil. With a spoon remove any fat floating on the surface. Add the rosemary branch. Pour in the sauce from the acorn and figs. Bring to boil and reduce to approximately 1 cup. If necessary, thicken with a little cornstarch and water mixture and bring to a boil. Add the parsley, any rendered meat juices, and bring to a boil. Adjust seasonings.

Slice the roast and place in a serving platter. Add the acorn squash and figs around the roast. Pour the sauce over the meat, sprinkle the almonds over the vegetables, and serve immediately.

The pork and figs may be refrigerated separately up to 5 days.

Freezing is not recommended for the figs and acorn squash. The pork and its sauce may be frozen up to 1 month.

Wine Suggestion: Viognier or a medium German Riesling or Gewürztraminer.

SERVING SIZE: One 5-ounce loin pork roast

PER SERVING: 510 Cal (22% from Fat, 28% from Protein, 50% from Carb); 36 g Protein; 13 g Tot Fat; 4 g Sat Fat; 6 g Mono Fat; 64 g Carb; 9 g Fiber; 30 g Sugar; 170 mg Calcium; 4 mg Iron; 195 mg Sodium; 78 mg Cholesterol

YIELD: 4 servings

Petits Poulets aux Olives
(Cornish Hen with Olives)

Preheat the oven to 350 degrees F.

Make a small X incision on the top and bottom of the tomatoes. Blanch the tomatoes for 20 seconds. Place in ice-cold water to stop the cooking process. Peel, seed, and dice the tomatoes.

Wash and pat dry the inside and outside of the Cornish hens. Place the hens in a baking pan, brush them with oil, and sprinkle with pepper. Add the onions, tomatoes, garlic, wine, and herbs de Provence to the pan. Bake for 1 hour. If the vegetables get too dry during the cooking process, add some chicken stock.

Meanwhile, cook the rice according to package directions.

2 Cornish hens
1 tablespoon olive oil
1 pound tomatoes (about 3 large tomatoes, diced small)
4 ounces onions, diced small (about 1 small onion)
3 garlic cloves, minced
6 ounces green olives, pitted
1/4 cup Chardonnay
1/2 cup chicken stock (low-fat and low-sodium)
1/2 teaspoon herbs de Provence
2 tablespoons fresh basil, minced
Salt and pepper to taste
1/2 cup rice

Remove the hens from the pan and set aside in a serving platter. Cover with aluminum foil to keep warm. Transfer the sauce to a saucepan. If the sauce is too dry, add more chicken stock. Add the olives, basil, and bring to a boil. Pour the sauce over the hens and serve immediately with the rice.

The hens and rice may be refrigerated separately up to 5 days.

The hens and rice may be frozen separately up to 1 month.

Note: If you must, you can substitute a small chicken, quartered for the Cornish hens, but I don't recommend it because the cooking times will really vary depending upon the size of the pieces.

Wine Suggestion: Chardonnay.

SERVING SIZE: 1/2 Cornish hen

PER SERVING: 490 Cal (60% from Fat, 26% from Protein, 14% from Carb); 31 g Protein; 32 g Tot Fat; 8 g Sat Fat; 16 g Mono Fat; 17 g Carb; 3 g Fiber; 1 g Sugar; 81 mg Calcium; 4 mg Iron; 521 mg Sodium; 170 mg Cholesterol

YIELD: 4 servings

Oie Farcie aux Marrons
(ROASTED GOOSE WITH CHESTNUTS)

FOR THE GOOSE:

6 to 7 pounds goose

2 pounds chestnuts

12 ounces apples, peeled, cored, diced small, and mixed with a little lemon juice (about 2 large apples)

8 ounces celery stalks, diced small (about 4 large celery stalks)

4 cups chicken stock (low-fat and low-sodium)

1/2 teaspoon dried thyme

1/2 teaspoon dried marjoram

4 tablespoons fresh parsley, minced

2 teaspoons salt

1/2 teaspoon pepper

Cornstarch plus water

1 tablespoon canola oil

Twine

For the goose: Slit the chestnut shells and place them in a pan. Cover with water and bring to a boil. Simmer for 2 minutes and remove from heat. Let cool a bit and then start removing one chestnut at a time to peel them. Place the peeled chestnuts in a saucepan and add enough chicken stock to cover them. Bring to a boil over high heat. Cover, reduce heat, and cook for 20 minutes or until barely tender. Strain the chestnuts keeping the stock for later use.

Preheat the oven to 350 degrees F.

In a bowl, mix the chestnuts, apples, and celery. Add the thyme, marjoram, parsley, salt, and pepper. Mix well and stuff the goose with this mixture. Close the opening tight with twine. Place the goose on a rack over a roasting pan. Add 1 cup water to the pan. Rub the goose with canola oil and roast for 2 1/2 to 3 hours or until done. Baste the goose every 20 minutes and add water in the pan, as it evaporates during the cooking process.

Remove from the oven and transfer the goose to a serving platter. Cover with aluminum foil to keep warm. Add 1 1/2 cups stock and scrape the particles from the bottom of the pan. Transfer to a saucepan and bring to a boil over high heat. With a spoon remove any fat floating on the surface. Reduce the sauce to concentrate its flavors. Thicken with a little cornstarch and water mixture, bring to a boil, and adjust seasonings.

Spoon out the goose stuffing into a serving bowl. Slice the goose and place on a serving platter. Pour over a little bit of the sauce and place the remaining sauce in a sauceboat. Serve immediately with the watercress and the stuffing.

For the watercress: In a bowl mix the oil, lemon juice, mustard, fines herbes, and season to taste. Top with the watercress but do not mix until serving time.

This recipe can also be done with turkey.

Chef's Tip: The amount of cornstarch and water mixture may vary depending on the amount of water rendered by the goose and the reduction process. To obtain the right thickness for a sauce: Dip a spoon in the sauce, turn it over, and make a line across with your finger. Tilt the spoon. If the sauce does not run over the line, it is the perfect thickness. If it does, you need to thicken with a little cornstarch and water mixture. After adding them, you will need to bring the sauce to a boil. Also, if it gets too thick, just add a little liquid to thin out.

FOR THE WATERCRESS:

3 large bunches watercress, washed and pat dry

3 tablespoons sunflower oil

1 tablespoon lemon juice

1 tablespoon fines herbes

1 teaspoon mustard

Salt and pepper to taste

Chef's Tip: To remove fat from a sauce, bring the sauce to boil and move half of the pan off the fire. The fat and the sauce will separate. The fat will be concentrated on one side of the pan making it easy to remove with a spoon. Doing this will considerably reduce the amount of fat in your recipe and therefore the final calorie count.

Chef's Secret: Add a little demi-glace (or demiglaze) to emphasize the sauce flavors. Demi-glace is a highly concentrated rich brown sauce that has been reduced by half. It is easily found in powder or paste form in grocery stores, in specialty stores, or over the Internet. It really adds tremendous flavor to finish a sauce without the fat you would get with butter.

Wine Suggestion: Riesling, Beaujolais, Haut-Médoc, Médoc, Gevrey Chambertin, or Pomerol.

SERVING SIZE: 5 ounces of goose meat without skin

PER SERVING: 495 Cal (50% from Fat, 21% from Protein, 29% from Carb); 26 g Protein; 28 g Tot Fat; 7 g Sat Fat; 12 g Mono Fat; 35 g Carb; 1 g Fiber; 4 g Sugar; 97 mg Calcium; 5 mg Iron; 897 mg Sodium; 86 mg Cholesterol

YIELD: 8 to 10 servings

Civet de Lapin à la Grecque
(RABBIT STEW GREEK STYLE)

Blanch the pearl onions in boiling water for 2 minutes. Let cool, peel, and set aside. Dredge the rabbit pieces in the flour. Shake off excess flour.

Heat half of the olive oil in a large nonstick pan over high heat. Add half of the rabbit pieces and brown on both sides. Remove and set aside in a deep pan. Repeat the process with the remaining pieces.

Deglaze the pan with a little stock and pour over the rabbit pieces. To deglaze, add a liquid (such as wine, stock, or water) and swirl to dissolve cooked particles on the bottom or side of the pan. Add 1 teaspoon olive oil to the deglazed pan, add the pearl onions, and cook until slightly browned over medium heat. Transfer to the rabbit pan. Add the garlic, wine, stock, lemon juice, and bouquet garni to the rabbit pan. Cover and simmer for 15 minutes. Add the potatoes, mushrooms, and continue to cook for 15 minutes or until the potatoes are tender.

3 pounds rabbit (or chicken), cut into individual portions
3 tablespoons flour
4 teaspoons olive oil
3 garlic cloves, minced
1 pound pearl onions
1 1/2 cups Chardonnay wine (lemony and buttery)
1 1/2 cups chicken stock (low-fat and low-sodium)
1 lemon, juiced
1 bouquet garni
3 tablespoons fresh parsley, minced
8 ounces white mushrooms (about 8 mushrooms)
12 small white potatoes, peeled (about 1 pound)
Salt and pepper to taste

Transfer the rabbit pieces, potatoes, and vegetables to a serving platter. Cover with aluminum foil to keep warm. Discard the bouquet garni. With a spoon remove any fat floating on the surface of the sauce. Reduce the sauce a little more to concentrate its flavors. If necessary, thicken with a little cornstarch and water mixture. Add the parsley and adjust seasonings. Pour over the rabbit and serve immediately.

The stew may be refrigerated up to 5 days.

The stew may be frozen up to 1 month.

Chef's Tip: The amount of cornstarch and water mixture may vary depending on the amount of water rendered by the rabbit and the reduction process. To obtain the right thickness for a sauce: Dip a spoon in the sauce, turn it over, and make a line across with your finger. Tilt the spoon. If the sauce does not run over the line, it is the perfect thickness. If it does, you need to thicken with a little cornstarch and water mixture. After adding them, you will need to bring the sauce to a boil. Also, if it gets too thick, just add a little liquid to thin out.

Chef's Tip: To remove fat from a sauce, bring the sauce to boil and move half of the pan off the fire. The fat and the sauce will separate. The fat will be concentrated on one side of the pan making it easy to remove with a spoon. Doing this will considerably reduce the amount of fat in your recipe and therefore the final calorie count.

Chef's Secret: Add a little demi-glace (or demiglaze) to emphasize the sauce flavors. Demi-glace is a highly concentrated rich brown sauce that has been reduced by half. It is easily found in powder or paste form in grocery stores, in specialty stores, or over the Internet. It really adds tremendous flavor to finish a sauce without the fat you would get with butter.

Wine Suggestion: Chardonnay (lemony and buttery).

SERVING SIZE 4 ounces rabbit

PER SERVING: 444 Cal (20% from Fat, 54% from Protein, 26% from Carb); 54 g Protein; 9 g Tot Fat; 2 g Sat Fat; 4 g Mono Fat; 26 g Carb; 4 g Fiber; 5 g Sugar; 70 mg Calcium; 9 mg Iron; 265 mg Sodium; 184 mg Cholesterol

YIELD: 6 servings

CHAPTER

4

Soups and Salads

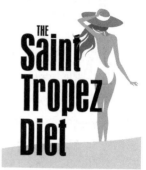

Gazpacho

Soak the bread in cold water for 5 minutes. Place all the ingredients in a blender. Mix until smooth. Add salt and cayenne pepper to taste. Refrigerate and serve cold.

The gazpacho may be refrigerated 2 to 3 days.

The gazpacho may be frozen up to 1 month.

SERVING SIZE: about 6 ounces

PER SERVING: 172 Cal (51% from Fat, 7% from Protein, 42% from Carb); 3 g Protein; 10 g Tot Fat; 1 g Sat Fat; 7 g Mono Fat; 19 g Carb; 3 g Fiber; 4 g Sugar; 37 mg Calcium; 1 mg Iron; 211 mg Sodium; 0 mg Cholesterol

YIELD: 12 servings

4 slices of bread

4 ounces olive oil

2 1/2 pounds tomatoes, diced (about 7 large tomatoes)

1 pound cucumbers, diced (about 2 medium cucumbers)

8 ounces onions, diced (about 1 large onion)

4 ounces green peppers, diced (about 1 medium green pepper)

6 garlic cloves, chopped

2 cups tomato juice

2 ounces red wine vinegar

2 tablespoons fresh basil, chopped

1 tablespoon fresh tarragon, chopped

Dash ground cumin

Dash hot sauce

1 lemon, juiced

Salt and cayenne pepper to taste

Zuppa Di Ceci e Riso
(CHICKPEA, TOMATO, AND RICE SOUP)

Heat the oil in a large pan over high heat. Add the onions and sauté until translucent. Add the garlic, tomatoes, rosemary, and cook until the juices are evaporated. Add the rice, stock, and bring to boil. Reduce heat, cover, and simmer for 15 minutes. Add the chickpeas and continue to cook for 5 minutes. Add the parsley, season to taste, and serve immediately.

The soup may be refrigerated for 5 days.

The soup may be frozen up to 1 month.

SERVING SIZE: 8 ounces

PER SERVING: 391 Cal (15% from Fat, 22% from Protein, 64% from Carb); 22 g Protein; 6 g Tot Fat; 1 g Sat Fat; 2 g Mono Fat; 64 g Carb; 16 g Fiber; 12 g Sugar; 136 mg Calcium; 7 mg Iron; 719 mg Sodium; 0 mg Cholesterol

YIELD: 4 servings

1 teaspoon olive oil

4 ounces onions, diced (about 1 small onion)

8 ounces chopped Italian plum tomatoes (canned)

3 ounces uncooked rice (about 1/2 cup uncooked rice)

12 ounces cooked chickpeas

2 to 3 garlic cloves, minced

5 cups chicken stock (low-fat and low-sodium)

1/2 teaspoon fresh rosemary, minced

2 tablespoons fresh parsley, chopped

Salt and pepper to taste

Soupe de Potiron
(Pumpkin Soup)

Peel the pumpkin and cut the flesh into medium cubes.

Heat the oil in a large pan over high heat. Add the onions and sauté until translucent. Add the pumpkin, garlic, stock, milk, sage, and bring to boil. Reduce heat, cover, and simmer for 30 minutes. Purée in a blender using enough liquid to obtain a creamy consistency. Return to pan and season to taste. Before serving, add the yogurt, and garnish with the pumpkin seeds.

The soup may be refrigerated for 5 days (without yogurt).

The soup may be frozen up to 1 month (without yogurt).

1 teaspoon olive oil

3 pounds pumpkin

1 pound onions, sliced (about 2 large onions)

1 garlic clove, minced

6 cups chicken stock (low-fat and low-sodium)

2 cups milk

2 fresh sage leaves

6 tablespoons low-fat yogurt

2 tablespoons pumpkin seeds

Salt and pepper to taste

Serving size: 8 ounces

Per Serving: 183 Cal (12% from Fat, 21% from Protein, 67% from Carb); 10 g Protein; 3 g Tot Fat; 1 g Sat Fat; 1 g Mono Fat; 33 g Carb; 8 g Fiber; 16 g Sugar; 221 mg Calcium; 4 mg Iron; 615 mg Sodium; 5 mg Cholesterol

Yield: 6 servings

Soupe de Poisson
(FISH SOUP)

Make a small X incision on the top and bottom of the tomatoes. Blanch the tomatoes for 20 seconds. Remove and place the tomatoes in ice-cold water to stop the cooking process. Peel, seed, and dice the tomatoes. Set aside.

Heat the oil in a large pan over high heat. Add the onions and sauté until translucent. Add the carrots, garlic, and sauté for 2 minutes. Add the wine and reduce by half. Add the stock, bouquet garni, tomatoes, parsley, orange zest, saffron, fennel seeds, and bring to a boil. Reduce heat, add the fish, and simmer until the fish starts to flake. Remove the bouquet garni and orange zest. Skim the surface, adjust seasonings, and serve immediately.

For this soup, these fish work best: cod, seabream, eel, haddock, hake, mackerel, monkfish, perch, red snapper, or white fish. Remember, the total calories will vary depending on the fish selected.

The soup may be refrigerated for 2 days.

The soup may be frozen up to 1 month.

2 teaspoons olive oil

8 ounces onions, diced small (about 1 large onion)

4 ounces carrots, diced small (about 1 large carrot)

5 garlic cloves, minced

6 ounces Chardonnay (or other wine with citrus and buttery flavor)

5 pounds various fish (see note below)

6 cups fish stock (low-sodium)

1 bouquet garni

1/2 pound tomatoes (about 2 medium tomatoes)

1/4 cup fresh parsley, minced

1 large strip orange zest

4 saffron sprigs

1 teaspoon fennel seeds

Salt and pepper to taste

SERVING SIZE: 6 to 8 ounces

PER SERVING (AVERAGE): 486 Cal (17% from Fat, 75% from Protein, 9% from Carb); 84 g Protein; 8 g Tot Fat; 2 g Sat Fat; 2 g Mono Fat; 10 g Carb; 2 g Fiber; 3 g Sugar; 224 mg Calcium; 2 mg Iron; 1039 mg Sodium; 140 mg Cholesterol

YIELD: 6 to 8 servings

Soupe de Lentilles
(LENTIL SOUP)

Heat the oil in a large pan over high heat. Add the onions and sauté until translucent. Add the carrot, celery, garlic, and cook for 2 minutes. Add the stock, ham bone, lentils, bouquet garni, and bring to a boil. Reduce heat, cover, and simmer for 35 minutes. Skim the surface as needed. Continue to simmer uncovered for 10 minutes to thicken the soup. Remove any fat that may rise to the surface of the soup. Remove the ham bone and bouquet garni. Adjust seasonings and serve immediately.

If the soup turns out too thick, adjust with stock. If the soup is too thin, reduce the liquid more.

2 teaspoons canola oil

8 ounces onions, diced small (about 1 large onion)

4 ounces carrots, diced small (about 1 large carrot)

4 ounces celery stalks, diced small (about 2 large celery stalks)

2 garlic cloves, minced

6 cups chicken stock (low-fat and low-sodium)

1 small ham bone (option)

12 ounces dried lentils (about 3 cups)

1 bouquet garni

Salt and pepper to taste

The soup may be refrigerated up to 5 days.

The soup may be frozen up to 1 month.

Chicken stock may be substituted with vegetable stock.

SERVING SIZE: 6 to 8 ounces

PER SERVING: 184 Cal (13% from Fat, 28% from Protein, 59% from Carb); 14 g Protein; 3 g Tot Fat; 0 g Sat Fat; 1 g Mono Fat; 28 g Carb; 9 g Fiber; 6 g Sugar; 79 mg Calcium; 4 mg Iron; 877 mg Sodium; 0 mg Cholesterol

YIELD: 4 to 6 servings

Soupe de Champignons aux Noisettes
(MUSHROOM AND HAZELNUT SOUP)

Heat the oil in a large pan over high heat. Add the onions and sauté until translucent. Add the mushrooms and cook for 2 minutes. Add the stock, potatoes, and bring to a boil. Reduce heat and simmer for 15 minutes. Purée in a blender with just enough stock to obtain a creamy consistency. Add the chives and season to taste.

Before serving add the yogurt. Do not boil or the yogurt will curdle. Garnish with the hazelnuts and serve immediately.

The soup may be refrigerated up to 5 days (without yogurt).

The soup may be frozen up to 1 month (without yogurt).

Chicken stock may be substituted with vegetable stock.

1 teaspoon canola oil
1 1/2 pounds mushrooms, sliced, any kind (about 24 small or 12 large mushrooms)
4 ounces onions, sliced thinly (about 1 small onion)
5 to 6 cups chicken stock (low-fat and low-sodium)
4 ounces potatoes, skin removed and diced small (about 1 medium potato)
2 tablespoons chives, minced
4 tablespoons low-fat yogurt
4 ounces hazelnuts, chopped (about 1 cup)
Salt and pepper to taste

SERVING SIZE: About 6 ounces

PER SERVING: 293 Cal (57% from Fat, 18% from Protein, 25% from Carb); 14 g Protein; 20 g Tot Fat; 2 g Sat Fat; 15 g Mono Fat; 20 g Carb; 6 g Fiber; 7 g Sugar; 102 mg Calcium; 3 mg Iron; 998 mg Sodium; 1 mg Cholesterol

YIELD: 4 servings

Soupe au Pistou
(SOUP WITH PISTOU)

For the soup: Chop the vegetables into equal sizes.

Place the white and red beans in a pan and cover with water. Bring to a boil over high heat. Remove from heat and set aside for 1 hour.

Heat some water, a pinch of salt, and a dash of oil over high heat. When boiling, add the pasta and cook until al dente. Strain, mix in a little oil, and set aside.

Make a small X incision on the top and bottom of the tomatoes. Blanch them for 20 seconds in the boiling water. Remove and place in ice-cold water to stop the cooking process. Remove the skin, seed, and chop.

Bring to a boil 10 cups of water in a large pan. Heat the oil in a large stockpot over high heat. Add the onions and sauté until translucent. Add the leeks, garlic, tomatoes, and cook for 5 minutes. Add the remaining ingredients (except pasta), 8 to 10 cups of the prepared water (enough to cover), and bring to a boil. Reduce heat, cover, and simmer for 1 hour or until the beans are cooked through. Mash the potatoes with a fork to thicken the soup.

FOR THE SOUP:

1 tablespoon olive oil

6 ounces white beans (about 1cup)

6 ounces red beans (about 1 cup)

6 ounces green beans, trimmed and cut into bite-sized pieces

6 ounces leeks, chopped (about 1 medium leek)

6 ounces zucchini, chopped (about 1 large zucchini)

8 ounces onions, chopped (about 1 large onion)

6 ounces carrots, chopped (about 2 medium carrots)

1 pound potatoes, skin removed and chopped (about 2 large potatoes)

1 pound tomatoes (about 3 large tomatoes)

6 garlic cloves, minced

1/4 cup fresh parsley, chopped

2 sage leaves

3 ounces whole wheat penne pasta (about 1 cup)

Salt and pepper to taste

FOR THE PISTOU:

6 garlic cloves

1 cup fresh basil

2 ounces Parmesan cheese

2 ounces olive oil

Adjust seasonings and add the pasta. Serve immediately with the pistou.

For the pistou: In a food processor mix the garlic, basil, Parmesan cheese, and a little oil. Slowly add the remaining oil. If the mixture is too thick, thin out with a little liquid from the soup.

The soup may be refrigerated up to 5 days.

The soup may be frozen up to 1 month.

SERVING SIZE: about 8 ounces

PER SERVING: 512 Cal (27% from Fat, 16% from Protein, 57% from Carb); 21 g Protein; 16 g Tot Fat; 3 g Sat Fat; 10 g Mono Fat; 76 g Carb; 15 g Fiber; 7 g Sugar; 260 mg Calcium; 7 mg Iron; 331 mg Sodium; 8 mg Cholesterol

YIELD: 6 servings

Soupe de Carottes à l'Orange
(CARROT AND ORANGE SOUP)

Juice three oranges and set aside. Dice the remaining oranges and set aside.

Heat the oil in a large pan over high heat. Add the onions and sauté until translucent. Add the carrots, garlic, and cook for 1 minute. Add the stock, potatoes, orange juice, coriander, ginger, honey, and bring to a boil. Reduce heat, cover, and simmer for 15 minutes. Purée the soup in a blender and return to pan. Add a little lemon juice, mint, and season to taste over low heat.

Before serving, mix in the yogurt. Do not boil or the yogurt will curdle. Add the diced oranges and serve immediately.

The soup may be refrigerated for 5 days (without yogurt).

The soup may be frozen up to 1 month (without yogurt).

Chicken stock may be substituted with vegetable stock.

1 teaspoon canola oil
4 ounces onions, minced (about 1 small onion)
1 pound carrots, shredded (about 4 large carrots)
1 garlic clove, minced
1/3 cup chicken stock (low-fat and low-sodium)
3 ounces potatoes, skin removed and shredded (about 1 small potato)
1 lemon
5 oranges
1/8 teaspoon ground coriander
1/2 tablespoon honey
1 teaspoon fresh ginger, minced
1 tablespoon fresh mint, minced
4 tablespoons low-fat yogurt
Salt and pepper to taste

SERVING SIZE: about 6 ounces

PER SERVING: 220 Cal (8% from Fat, 9% from Protein, 84% from Carb); 5 g Protein; 2 g Tot Fat; 0 g Sat Fat; 1 g Mono Fat; 50 g Carb; 10 g Fiber; 31 g Sugar; 175 mg Calcium; 1 mg Iron; 138 mg Sodium; 1 mg Cholesterol

YIELD: 4 servings

Soupe de Betteraves au Fenouil
(BEET AND FENNEL SOUP)

Heat the oil in a large pan over high heat. Add the onions and sauté until translucent. Add the carrots, celery, garlic, and sauté for 2 minutes. Add the beets, fennel, ginger, stock, orange juice, and bring to a boil. Reduce heat, cover, and simmer for 30 minutes. Using a blender, purée the soup adding enough stock to obtain the right consistency. Season to taste and refrigerate for 2 hours before serving.

The soup may be refrigerated up to 5 days.

The soup may be frozen up to 1 month.

Chicken stock may be substituted with vegetable stock.

1 teaspoon canola oil

5 beets, peeled, cored, and chopped

3 fennel bulbs, cored, stems removed, and chopped

8 ounces onions, diced (about 1 large onion)

2 ounces carrots, diced (about 1 small carrot)

2 ounces celery, diced (about 1 large celery stalk)

1 garlic clove, minced

1 tablespoon fresh ginger, minced

5 to 6 cups chicken stock (low-fat and low-sodium)

2 tablespoons fresh orange juice

Salt and pepper to taste

SERVING SIZE: about 8 ounces

PER SERVING: 118 Cal (11% from Fat, 23% from Protein, 66% from Carb); 7 g Protein; 2 g Tot Fat; 0 g Sat Fat; 1 g Mono Fat; 21 g Carb; 7 g Fiber; 4 g Sugar; 160 mg Calcium; 3 mg Iron; 874 mg Sodium; 0 mg Cholesterol

YIELD: 4 servings

Soupe à l'Oignon
(ONION SOUP)

Heat the oil in a large pan over medium heat. Add the onions and cook until golden brown.Stir occasionally to avoid burning. This will take up to 20 minutes. Carefully add the cognac and flambé. Sprinkle the flour and mix well. Add the beef stock and bring to a boil over high heat. Reduce heat and simmer for 20 to 25 minutes. Skim any foam or fat that rises to the surface. Adjust seasonings and serve immediately.

2 tablespoons grapeseed oil
1 1/2 pounds onions, thinly
    sliced (about 3 large onions)
2 tablespoons cognac (optional)
2 tablespoons flour
6 to 7 cups beef stock (low-fat
    and low-sodium)
Salt and pepper to taste

The soup may be refrigerated for 5 days.

The soup may be frozen up to 1 month.

Beef stock can be substituted with vegetable stock.

SERVING SIZE: 6 to 8 ounces

PER SERVING: 187 Cal (40% from Fat, 14% from Protein, 46% from Carb); 6 g Protein; 8 g Tot Fat; 1 g Sat Fat; 1 g Mono Fat; 20 g Carb; 2 g Fiber; 7 g Sugar; 60 mg Calcium; 1 mg Iron; 1179 mg Sodium; 0 mg Cholesterol

YIELD: 4 to 6 servings

Melon aux Figues et Prosciutto
(MELON WITH FIGS AND PROSCIUTTO)

Boil the pomegranate vinegar over high heat. Reduce by half and cool down. Refrigerate before use.

Cut the cantaloupe in half. Scoop out the seeds and drain any liquid. Cut each half into half again and remove skin. Remove the figs skins and cut in half.

Place one melon wedge on a plate. Add one Prosciutto slice and 2 fig halves. Sprinkle with some vinegar, pepper, and serve immediately.

1 large cantaloupe

4 slices Prosciutto

4 fresh figs

1/2 cup pomegranate or
    balsamic vinegar

Pepper to taste

SERVING SIZE: 1/4 cantaloupe, 1 Prosciutto slice, 1 fig, and 1 tablespoon pomegranate vinegar.

PER SERVING: 223 Cal (24% from Fat, 36% from Protein, 41% from Carb); 20 g Protein; 6 g Tot Fat; 2 g Sat Fat; 3 g Mono Fat; 23 g Carb; 3 g Fiber; 21 g Sugar; 33 mg Calcium; 1 mg Iron; 1858 mg Sodium; 48 mg Cholesterol

YIELD: 4 servings

Salade de Canard Fumé à la Vinaigrette de Framboise
(Smoked Duck Salad with Raspberry Vinaigrette)

For the vinaigrette: In a large bowl combine the vinegars, mustard, shallot, and preserves. Mix thoroughly and slowly whisk in the oils. Add the herbs and season to taste. If it is too tart for your taste, add a little more preserves.

For the salad: Using a sharp knife, thinly slice the duck breasts and sprinkle pepper. In a bowl, mix the mesclun greens with 3/4 of the dressing. Transfer the mesclun greens to a serving platter. Add the duck slices, glazed walnuts, and berries. Drizzle the remaining dressing and serve immediately.

FOR THE SALAD:

10 ounces smoked duck breast

5 ounces mesclun greens

1 cup raspberries, cleaned and pat dry

1/4 cup glazed walnuts

FOR THE VINAIGRETTE:

2 tablespoons raspberry vinegar

1 tablespoon pomegranate vinegar

1/2 teaspoon Dijon mustard

1 large shallot, minced

4 tablespoons olive oil

2 tablespoons walnut oil

1 tablespoon seedless currant preserves

2 tablespoons fresh salad herbs

Salt and pepper to taste

Serving size: 1/4 recipe

Per Serving: 410 Cal (71% from Fat, 19% from Protein, 10% from Carb); 20 g Protein; 33 g Tot Fat; 5 g Sat Fat; 18 g Mono Fat; 10 g Carb; 3 g Fiber; 5 g Sugar; 36 mg Calcium; 3 mg Iron; 80 mg Sodium; 96 mg Cholesterol

Yield: 4 servings

Salade d'Artichauds et de Fèves
(ARTICHOKES AND FAVA BEANS SALAD)

For the vinaigrette: In a bowl mix the shallots, garlic, mustard, and vinegar. Slowly whisk in the oils. Add the herbs and season to taste.

For the salad: Line a serving platter with the lettuce. Spread the fava beans, artichoke hearts, and tomatoes on top of the lettuce. Drizzle with the vinaigrette. Add the feta cheese, almonds, and serve immediately.

If fava beans are unavailable, use butter beans, broad beans, windsor beans, or lima beans.

FOR THE SALAD:

8 ounces cooked fava beans

1 cup cooked artichoke hearts

8 cherry tomatoes

4 ounces Boston lettuce

4 ounces feta cheese, cut into 1 inch cubes

4 teaspoons slivered almonds

FOR THE VINAIGRETTE:

2 shallots, minced

1 large garlic clove, minced

1 teaspoon Dijon mustard

4 tablespoons balsamic vinegar

6 tablespoons olive oil

2 tablespoons flaxseed oil

3 tablespoons fresh salad herbs, minced

Salt and pepper to taste

SERVING SIZE: 1/4 Artichokes and Fava Beans Salad

PER SERVING: 403 Cal (73% from Fat, 11% from Protein, 16% from Carb); 12 g Protein; 35 g Tot Fat; 8 g Sat Fat; 19 g Mono Fat; 18 g Carb; 3 g Fiber; 3 g Sugar; 176 mg Calcium; 1 mg Iron; 358 mg Sodium; 25 mg Cholesterol

YIELD: 4 servings

Poireaux à la Vinaigrette de Noix
(Leeks with Walnut Vinaigrette)

FOR THE SALAD:

8 small leeks

FOR THE VINAIGRETTE:

1 large garlic clove, minced

1 large shallot, minced

1 teaspoon Dijon mustard

4 tablespoons walnut oil

2 tablespoons olive oil

2 tablespoons tarragon vinegar

1/4 cup walnuts, finely chopped

1 tablespoon fresh chives, minced

1 tablespoon fresh parsley, minced

Salt and pepper to taste

For the vinaigrette: In a bowl mix the garlic, shallot, mustard, walnuts, and vinegar. Slowly whisk in the oils. Add the chives, parsley, and season to taste.

For the leeks: Wash and trim the leeks. Place the leeks in a pan and cover with water. Bring to boil over high heat. Reduce heat, cover, and simmer for 10 minutes or until tender.

Strain and cut the leeks in half lengthwise. Mix the leeks with the vinaigrette and let cool. Refrigerate and serve cold.

SERVING SIZE: 2 leeks

PER SERVING: 286 Cal (77% from Fat, 4% from Protein, 20% from Carb); 3 g Protein; 25 g Tot Fat; 4 g Sat Fat; 12 g Mono Fat; 15 g Carb; 2 g Fiber; 4 g Sugar; 63 mg Calcium; 2 mg Iron; 33 mg Sodium; 0 mg Cholesterol

YIELD: 4 servings

Tomates au Basilic
(Tomato and Basil Salad)

Discard each end of the tomatoes. Slice the tomatoes and spread them over a platter. Sprinkle with a little salt and set aside for 20 minutes.

In a bowl, mix the shallot, garlic, vinegar, and whisk in the oils. Add half of the basil, parsley, and season to taste.

Transfer the tomatoes to another serving platter. Spread the remaining basil, pour over the dressing, and serve immediately.

2 pounds tomatoes (about 6 large tomatoes)
1 shallot, minced
1 large garlic clove, minced
3 tablespoons olive oil
1 tablespoon flaxseed oil
2 tablespoons aged balsamic vinegar
6 to 8 fresh basil leaves, shredded
1 tablespoon fresh parsley, minced
Salt and pepper to taste

SERVING SIZE: 1/4 recipe

PER SERVING: 172 Cal (70% from Fat, 5% from Protein, 25% from Carb); 2 g Protein; 14 g Tot Fat; 2 g Sat Fat; 8 g Mono Fat; 12 g Carb; 3 g Fiber; 0 g Sugar; 17 mg Calcium; 1 mg Iron; 22 mg Sodium; 0 mg Cholesterol

YIELD: 4 servings

Salade de Carottes au Citron
(CARROT SALAD WITH LEMON)

FOR THE SALAD:
1 pound carrots (about 4 large carrots)
6 ounces apples (about 1 large apple)
4 teaspoons walnuts

FOR THE VINAIGRETTE:
1 large garlic clove, minced
1 teaspoon Dijon mustard
2 tablespoons canola oil
2 tablespoons flaxseed oil
2 tablespoons lemon juice
1 tablespoon parsley, minced
Salt and pepper to taste

For the vinaigrette: In a bowl mix the garlic, mustard, and lemon juice. Blend in the oils. Add the parsley and season to taste.

For the salad: Peel and shred the carrots, and immediately mix with the vinaigrette. Peel, core, and shred the apples, and immediately add to the carrots. Blend well and adjust seasonings. Add the walnuts and serve immediately.

SERVING SIZE: 1/4 recipe

PER SERVING: 210 Cal (64% from Fat, 3% from Protein, 33% from Carb); 2 g Protein; 16 g Tot Fat; 1 g Sat Fat; 6 g Mono Fat; 18 g Carb; 4 g Fiber; 10 g Sugar; 45 mg Calcium; 1 mg Iron; 93 mg Sodium; 0 mg Cholesterol

YIELD: 4 servings

Salade de Poulet au Céleri et Pomme
(Chicken Salad with Celery and Apple)

FOR THE SALAD:

6 ounces Romaine heart leaves, chopped (about 1 large head of Romaine heart leaves)

12 ounces cooked chicken breasts, diced

12 ounces apples (about 2 large apples)

4 ounces celery, diced (about 2 large celery stalks)

1/4 cup walnuts, chopped

1 lemon, juiced

FOR THE VINAIGRETTE:

2 tablespoons cider vinegar

1 tablespoon lemon juice

2 teaspoons honey

1 tablespoon walnut oil

2 tablespoons olive oil

2 tablespoons fresh parsley, chopped

Salt and pepper to taste

For the vinaigrette: In a large bowl mix the vinegar, 1 tablespoon lemon juice, honey, oil, parsley, and season to taste.

For the salad: Peel, core, and dice the apples. Mix them with some lemon juice to prevent browning. In a bowl, place the romaine, chicken, apples, and celery. Mix in the dressing, add the walnuts, and serve immediately.

SERVING SIZE: 1/4 recipe

PER SERVING: 304 Cal (49% from Fat, 24% from Protein, 26% from Carb); 20 g Protein; 18 g Tot Fat; 3 g Sat Fat; 8 g Mono Fat; 21 g Carb; 5 g Fiber; 13 g Sugar; 61 mg Calcium; 2 mg Iron; 83 mg Sodium; 55 mg Cholesterol

YIELD: 4 servings

Salade du Pêcheur
(FISHERMAN SALAD)

FOR THE SALAD:

12 ounces salmon (canned in water)

3 3/4 ounces sardines (canned in oil)

5 ounces baby lettuce mix

12 ounces tomatoes, sliced (about 2 large tomatoes)

6 ounces cooked artichoke hearts,
  quartered (about 3/4 cup artichoke hearts)

6 ounces green bell peppers, seeded, ribs
  removed, and chopped (about 1 large green
  bell pepper)

2 tablespoons scallions, chopped

4 ounces cucumber, halved and sliced (about 1/2
  medium cucumber)

2 ounces white mushrooms, sliced (about 2 white
  mushrooms)

FOR THE DRESSING:

1 teaspoon Dijon mustard

1 tablespoon shallot, minced

1 teaspoon garlic, minced

2 tablespoons wine vinegar

1 tablespoon lemon juice

5 tablespoons olive oil

2 teaspoons fresh dill, minced

1 tablespoon fresh parsley, minced

2 teaspoons fresh tarragon, minced

Salt and pepper to taste

For the dressing: In a bowl, mix the mustard, shallots, garlic, vinegar, and lemon juice. Slowly whisk in the oil. Blend in the herbs and season to taste.

For the salad: In a large bowl, place the lettuce, tomatoes, artichoke hearts, green bell peppers, scallions, cucumber, and mushrooms. Mix in the vinaigrette, add the salmon, sardines, and serve immediately.

SERVING SIZE: 1/4 recipe

PER SERVING: 409 Cal (55% from Fat, 28% from Protein, 16% from Carb); 30 g Protein; 26 g Tot Fat; 4 g Sat Fat; 15 g Mono Fat; 17 g Carb; 6 g Fiber; 4 g Sugar; 376 mg Calcium; 3 mg Iron; 320 mg Sodium; 73 mg Cholesterol

YIELD: 4 servings

Salade Niçoise
(Niçoise Salad)

For the dressing: In a bowl, mix the shallot, garlic, mustard, vinegar, oils, 2 tablespoons herbs, anchovy fillets, and a pinch of pepper. Purée with a hand blender. If too thick, add a little water to thin out. Taste and adjust seasonings.

For the salad: Place the eggs in a pan, cover with cold water, add 2 teaspoons salt, and bring to a boil over medium heat. Reduce heat and simmer for 10 minutes. Remove the eggs and place them in cold water. Peel, quarter, and set aside.

In a large bowl, mix the mixed greens with 3/4 of the dressing. Add the tomatoes, potatoes, bell peppers, cucumber, and green beans. Top with the tuna, eggs, and sprinkle with the remaining herbs. Drizzle with the remaining dressing and serve immediately.

SALAD:

5 ounces mixed greens

6 ounces canned tuna in water, strained

2 large tomatoes, seeded and diced

2 cooked medium potatoes, sliced

1 green bell pepper, seeded, ribs removed, and julienned

1 small cucumber, peeled and sliced

4 ounces cooked green beans, cut in half

2 ounces small niçoise black olives

4 eggs

DRESSING:

1 shallot, minced

1 garlic clove, minced

1 teaspoon Dijon mustard

2 tablespoons wine vinegar

4 tablespoons olive oil

2 tablespoons walnut oil

3 tablespoons fines herbs (salad herbs)

2 anchovy fillets

Salt and pepper to taste

Serving Size: 1/4 recipe

Per Serving: 560 Cal (56% from Fat, 20% from Protein, 25% from Carb); 28 g Protein; 35 g Tot Fat; 8 g Sat Fat; 19 g Mono Fat; 35 g Carb; 6 g Fiber; 3 g Sugar; 112 mg Calcium; 5 mg Iron; 550 mg Sodium; 272 mg Cholesterol

Yield: 4 servings

Salade Verte au Fromage de Chèvre
(MESCLUN GREENS WITH GOAT CHEESE)

For the vinaigrette: In a bowl, mix the mustard, garlic, shallot, and vinegar. Whisk in the oil, herbs, and season to taste.

For the salad: Place the mesclun greens in a bowl and mix in 3/4 of the vinaigrette. Crumb the goat cheese over the greens. Add the walnuts and dates. Drizzle with the remaining dressing and serve immediately.

Note: Medjool dates are a popular palm date variety throughout the world. It is one of the best and easy to find.

FOR THE SALAD:

6 ounces mesclun greens

4 ounces goat cheese

1/4 cup walnuts, chopped

8 Medjool dates

FOR THE VINAIGRETTE:

4 tablespoons olive oil

2 tablespoons walnut oil

1 teaspoon Dijon mustard

1 large garlic clove, minced

1 large shallot, minced

2 tablespoons Xères or sherry vinegar

2 tablespoons fresh fines herbs (or salad herbs)

Salt and pepper to taste

SERVING SIZE: 1/4 recipe

PER SERVING: 444 Cal (60% from Fat, 7% from Protein, 33% from Carb); 8 g Protein; 31 g Tot Fat; 8 g Sat Fat; 15 g Mono Fat; 39 g Carb; 4 g Fiber; 33 g Sugar; 97 mg Calcium; 2 mg Iron; 123 mg Sodium; 13 mg Cholesterol

YIELD: 4 servings

Salade Frisée à la Grecque
(CURLY ENDIVE GREEK STYLE)

For the dressing: In a bowl, mix the vinegar, oils, and garlic. Blend in the yogurt. Add the oregano, parsley, and season to taste.

For the salad: In a large bowl, place the curly endive, red onions, cucumbers, bell peppers, and tomatoes. Add the dressing and mix well. Add the olives, feta cheese, and serve immediately.

SERVING SIZE: 1/4 recipe

PER SERVING: 392 Cal (65% from Fat, 11% from Protein, 24% from Carb); 11 g Protein; 29 g Tot Fat; 8 g Sat Fat; 15 g Mono Fat; 25 g Carb; 4 g Fiber; 4 g Sugar; 162 mg Calcium; 3 mg Iron; 512 mg Sodium; 30 mg Cholesterol

YIELD: 4 servings

FOR THE SALAD:

1 head curly endive, cleaned and trimmed

4 ounces red onions, sliced (about 1 small red onion)

6 ounces cucumbers, sliced (about 1 medium cucumber)

6 ounces green bell peppers, sliced (about 1 large green bell pepper)

12 ounces tomatoes, sliced (about 2 large tomatoes)

1/2 cup feta cheese, crumbled

4 tablespoons black olives

FOR THE DRESSING:

2 tablespoons herb-flavored vinegar

4 tablespoons olive oil

1 tablespoon flaxseed oil

1 teaspoon garlic cloves, minced

2 tablespoons low-fat yogurt

1 tablespoon fresh oregano, minced

2 tablespoons fresh parsley, minced

Salt and pepper to taste

Salade de Lentilles
(LENTIL SALAD)

FOR THE SALAD:

1 pound lentils

1 tablespoon garlic cloves, minced

1 bouquet garni

1 bay leaf

1 orange, juiced

FOR THE DRESSING:

2 tablespoons wine vinegar

1 tablespoon shallot, minced

1 teaspoon Dijon mustard

6 tablespoons walnut oil

3 tablespoons fresh fines herbs
  (or salad herbs)

Salt and pepper to taste

For the dressing: In a bowl, mix the vinegar, shallot, and mustard. Slowly whisk in the oil. Add the herbs and season to taste.

For the salad: Rinse the lentils and place them in a pan. Add enough water to completely cover them. Bring to a boil over high heat. Remove from heat and set aside covered for 1 hour.

Strain and return to the large pan. Add water (3 times the volume of the lentils), garlic, bay leaf, and bouquet garni. Bring to a boil over high heat. Reduce heat, cover, and simmer for 20 to 25 minutes or until tender.

Remove the bouquet garni and bay leaf. Strain the lentils and transfer to a bowl. Mix in the vinaigrette and refrigerate for 30 minutes. Serve cold.

The lentils will keep refrigerated up to 5 days (without dressing).

The lentils will keep frozen up to 1 month (without dressing).

SERVING SIZE: 1/6 recipe

PER SERVING: 230 Cal (53% from Fat, 12% from Protein, 35% from Carb); 7 g Protein; 14 g Tot Fat; 2 g Sat Fat; 6 g Mono Fat; 21 g Carb; 7 g Fiber; 2 g Sugar; 40 mg Calcium; 3 mg Iron; 12 mg Sodium; 0 mg Cholesterol

YIELD: 6 servings

Salade de Calamars et Poivrons
(Squid and Roasted Bell Peppers Salad)

FOR THE SALAD:

1 teaspoon olive oil

1 pound squid, defrosted and rinsed

8 ounces red onions, thinly sliced (about
    1 large red onion)

3 red bell peppers

8 ounces cooked artichoke hearts (about
    1 cup cooked artichoke hearts)

12 pitted olives

FOR THE DRESSING:

1 large garlic clove, minced

3 tablespoons fresh basil, minced

1 tablespoon fresh parsley, minced

4 tablespoons olive oil

2 tablespoons flaxseed oil

3 tablespoons lemon juice

Salt and pepper to taste

For the dressing: In a bowl mix the garlic, olive oil, flaxseed oil, lemon juice, basil, parsley, and season to taste.

For the salad: Preheat the broiler. Place the red bell peppers on a baking sheet and char on all sides. If you have a gas stovetop, you may char the peppers over the flames. Once blackened, place them in a paper bag and seal. Let stand for 10 minutes. Peel the skin, remove ribs and seeds. Thinly slice and set aside.

Heat 1 teaspoon olive oil in a nonstick pan over medium heat. Add the squid and cook for 5 minutes or until slightly tender. Add the red onions and continue to cook for 2 to 3 minutes. Remove from heat and let cool. Transfer to a bowl. Add the bell peppers, artichoke hearts, and olives. Mix in the prepared dressing and refrigerate. Taste, adjust seasonings, and serve cold.

This salad may be served over lettuce.

SERVING SIZE: 1/4 recipe

PER SERVING: 393 Cal (56% from Fat, 21% from Protein, 23% from Carb); 21 g Protein; 25 g Tot Fat; 3 g Sat Fat; 13 g Mono Fat; 23 g Carb; 6 g Fiber; 8 g Sugar; 87 mg Calcium; 2 mg Iron; 200 mg Sodium; 264 mg Cholesterol

YIELD: 4 servings

Betteraves Rouges aux Noix
(BEETS WITH WALNUTS)

For the salad: Place the beets in a large pan and cover with water. Bring to boil over high heat. Reduce heat, cover, and simmer for 30 minutes or until tender. Strain and cool. Peel, slice the beets, and place in a serving bowl.

For the dressing: In a bowl mix the shallot, garlic, mustard, vinegar, lemon juice, and parsley. Blend in the oil and season to taste.

Mix the beets with the dressing, sprinkle the walnuts, and serve immediately.

This salad may be served over lettuce.

FOR THE SALAD:

20 ounces beets (about 2 large beets)

1/4 cup walnuts, chopped

FOR THE DRESSING:

1 small shallot, minced

1 large garlic clove, minced

1 teaspoon Dijon mustard

3 tablespoons walnut oil

1 1/2 tablespoons lemon juice

1 tablespoon fresh parsley, minced

Salt and pepper to taste

SERVING SIZE: 1/4 recipe

PER SERVING: 207 Cal (63% from Fat, 7% from Protein, 31% from Carb); 4 g Protein; 15 g Tot Fat; 2 g Sat Fat; 5 g Mono Fat; 17 g Carb; 5 g Fiber; 11 g Sugar; 34 mg Calcium; 1 mg Iron; 126 mg Sodium; 0 mg Cholesterol

YIELD: 4 servings

THE Saint Tropez Diet

Petits Poivrons Farcis au Thon
(Baby Bell Peppers with Tuna)

In a bowl mix the tuna, parsley, chives, and scallions. Sprinkle with a little bit of lemon juice. Mix in the mayonnaise and season to taste. Refrigerate until needed.

Cut off the tops of the bell peppers. Remove seeds and ribs. Fill with the tuna mixture and serve immediately.

The tuna mixture may be refrigerated 2 to 3 days.

24 baby bell peppers (approximately 4 cups)

12 ounces tuna (canned tuna in water)

2 tablespoons fresh parsley, minced

2 tablespoons fresh chives, minced

1/4 cup scallions, chopped small

1 lemon

6 tablespoons canola mayonnaise

Salt and pepper to taste

SERVING SIZE: 1 baby bell pepper

PER SERVING: 32 Cal (32% from Fat, 44% from Protein, 24% from Carb); 4 g Protein; 1 g Tot Fat; 0 g Sat Fat; 0 g Mono Fat; 2 g Carb; 0 g Fiber; 1 g Sugar; 7 mg Calcium; 0 mg Iron; 317 mg Sodium; 7 mg Cholesterol

YIELD: 24 servings

Tomato and Walnut Bruschetta

FOR THE BREAD:
1 french baguette

FOR THE BRUSCHETTA:
1 1/2 pounds Roma tomatoes (about 5 large Roma tomatoes)
3 ounces fresh mozzarella, chopped small
1/2 cup walnuts, chopped small
3 large garlic cloves, minced
1/3 cup fresh basil, chopped small
1 tablespoon fresh oregano, minced
2 tablespoons olive oil
1 tablespoon balsamic vinegar
1 teaspoon lemon juice
Salt and pepper to taste

Cut the tomatoes in half. Seed, dice, and place in a bowl. Add the remaining bruschetta ingredients and toss well. Refrigerate for a couple of hours.

Preheat the broiler. With a serrated knife cut the baguette into 1/2-inch thick slices. Place the slices on a baking sheet. Broil on both sides until golden brown. Cool before use.

Spoon some bruschetta mixture over each bread slice and serve immediately.

SERVING SIZE: 1 slice

PER SERVING: 47 Cal (61% from Fat, 15% from Protein, 24% from Carb); 2 g Protein; 3 g Tot Fat; 1 g Sat Fat; 1 g Mono Fat; 3 g Carb; 1 g Fiber; 1 g Sugar; 36 mg Calcium; 0 mg Iron; 37 mg Sodium; 2 mg Cholesterol

YIELD: 24 servings

Olive Paste and Red Bell Pepper Bruschetta

Preheat the broiler. Place the red bell peppers on a baking sheet and char on all sides. If you have a gas stovetop, you may char the bell peppers over the flames. Once blackened on all sides, place in a paper bag and seal. Let stand for 10 minutes. Peel and seed the bell peppers. Remove ribs and slice into 1/2-inch wide strips.

In a food processor purée the olives, capers, garlic, oil, lemon juice, and anchovy fillets. The paste should be smooth and spreadable. If it is too thick, add a little olive oil. Season to taste and refrigerate for 30 minutes.

Cut the baguette with a serrated knife into 3/4-inch thick slices. Place the slices on a baking sheet. Broil on both sides until golden brown. Cool before use.

Spread some olive paste on each bread slice and top with 1 slice of red bell pepper. Serve immediately.

The paste may be refrigerated up to 5 days. Cover the paste with a thin layer of olive oil to avoid dryness.

FOR THE BREAD:
1 french baguette

FOR THE BRUSCHETTA:
1 1/2 cups pitted black olives
2 ounces capers, rinsed and pat dry
4 large garlic cloves, minced
1/2 lemon, juiced
1/2 cup olive oil
2 ounces anchovy fillets, rinsed and pat dry
2 large red bell peppers
Salt and pepper to taste

SERVING SIZE: 1 slice

PER SERVING: 63 Cal (79% from Fat, 7% from Protein, 15% from Carb); 1 g Protein; 6 g Tot Fat; 1 g Sat Fat; 4 g Mono Fat; 2 g Carb; 1 g Fiber; 1 g Sugar; 16 mg Calcium; 1 mg Iron; 238 mg Sodium; 2 mg Cholesterol

YIELD: 24 servings

Pesto and Salmon Bruschetta

In a food processor purée the basil, parsley, lemon thyme, walnuts, garlic, 1 tablespoon lemon peel, and 1 tablespoon lemon juice. Gradually add the oil until you obtain a smooth paste. Add salt and pepper to taste. If too thick, add a little more oil.

Preheat the broiler. With a serrated knife cut the walnut bread into 1/2-inch thick slices. Cut each slice in half. Place the slices on a baking sheet. Broil on both sides until golden brown. Cool before using.

FOR THE BREAD:
1 loaf walnut bread

FOR THE BRUSCHETTA:
24 smoked salmon slices, rolled (about 1 pound, 2 ounces)
1 1/3 cup fresh basil
2/3 cup fresh parsley
2 tablespoons fresh lemon thyme, minced
1/2 cup walnuts
2 garlic cloves
1 lemon
1/4 cup olive oil
Salt and pepper to taste

Spread some pesto over each bread slice. Add one salmon roll, sprinkle each with a little lemon juice, and serve immediately.

The pesto may be refrigerated up to 5 days. Cover the pesto with a thin layer of olive oil to avoid dryness.

SERVING SIZE: 1 slice

PER SERVING: 76 Cal (55% from Fat, 25% from Protein, 20% from Carb); 5 g Protein; 5 g Tot Fat; 1 g Sat Fat; 2 g Mono Fat; 4 g Carb; 1 g Fiber; 0 g Sugar; 15 mg Calcium; 1 mg Iron; 179 mg Sodium; 4 mg Cholesterol

YIELD: 24 servings

Apple and Walnut Bruschetta

FOR THE BREAD:
1 loaf walnut bread

FOR THE BRUSCHETTA:
6 apples, washed and pat dry
Two 5-ounce goat cheese logs
1 fresh rosemary branch
1 tablespoon canola oil
6 tablespoons liquid honey
1/2 cup walnuts, chopped small
1 lemon, juiced
Pepper

Mince the rosemary as small as possible. Mix the lemon juice with the rosemary.

Peel, core, and quarter the apples. Slice each quarter into 3 slices. Place the apples in a bowl, mix in the flavored lemon juice, and set aside.

Heat the oil in a large sauté pan over high heat. Add the apples slices (without the lemon juice) and slightly brown. Remove the apples and set aside. The apples must be still slightly crunchy. Deglaze the pan with a little water and the remaining lemon juice. To deglaze, add a liquid (such as wine, stock, or water) and swirl to dissolve cooked particles on the bottom or side of the pan. Reduce to approximately 1 tablespoon. Strain while pouring over the apples and mix carefully.

Preheat the broiler. Cut the bread with a serrated knife into 3/4-inch thick slices. Cut each slice in half again. Place the slices on a baking sheet. Broil on both sides until golden brown. Cool before use.

Add 3 apple slices to each toasted bread slice. Lay on a thin slice of goat cheese and season to taste. Place under the broiler and slightly melt the cheese. Pour 1/4 teaspoon honey over each slice and sprinkle with walnuts. Serve immediately.

SERVING SIZE: 1 slice

Per Serving: 88 Cal (46% from Fat, 12% from Protein, 42% from Carb); 3 g Protein; 5 g Tot Fat; 2 g Sat Fat; 1 g Mono Fat; 10 g Carb; 1 g Fiber; 8 g Sugar; 23 mg Calcium; 0 mg Iron; 50 mg Sodium; 5 mg Cholesterol

YIELD: 24 servings

Champignons Fourrés à la Tapenade
(STUFFED MUSHROOMS WITH TAPENADE)

24 large mushrooms

1 cup pitted black olives

1 ounce capers, rinsed and pat dry

2 ounces anchovy fillets

4 garlic cloves, minced

3 ounces olive oil

1 teaspoon lemon juice

1 bunch fresh parsley, minced

Pepper

Preheat the broiler. Clean and empty the center part of each mushroom. Place the mushrooms on a baking sheet. Broil for 3 to 4 minutes until the mushrooms start to sweat. Do not overcook, as the mushrooms will start to shrink. Remove from the oven and set aside to cool down.

In a food processor purée the black olives, capers, anchovy, garlic, olive oil, and lemon juice. Add pepper to taste. Fill each mushroom with the tapenade, sprinkle with parsley, and serve immediately.

The tapenade may be refrigerated up to 5 days. Cover the tapenade with a thin layer of olive oil to avoid dryness.

SERVING SIZE: 1 mushroom

PER SERVING: 50 Cal (76% from Fat, 13% from Protein, 11% from Carb); 2 g Protein; 4 g Tot Fat; 1 g Sat Fat; 3 g Mono Fat; 1 g Carb; 1 g Fiber; 1 g Sugar; 12 mg Calcium; 0 mg Iron; 172 mg Sodium; 2 mg Cholesterol

YIELD: 24 servings

Lotte au Chutney de Noix
(MONKFISH WITH NUT CHUTNEY)

FOR THE FISH:

3 pounds thick monkfish fillets

1 garlic clove, minced

1/4 cup olive oil

3 tablespoons lime juice

1/4 teaspoon crushed hot red pepper flakes

24 small Romaine leaves

FOR THE CHUTNEY:

1 pound yogurt

1 teaspoon ground ginger

1 teaspoon ground coriander

1 teaspoon ground cumin

1 tablespoon olive oil

4 jalapeno chiles, minced

2 cups fresh cilantro, chopped

2 tablespoons lime juice

1/3 cup pistachios, chopped finely

1/3 cup walnuts, chopped finely

1/3 cup almonds, chopped finely

For the chutney: In a bowl mix the yogurt, ginger, coriander, cumin, olive oil, jalapenos, cilantro, lime juice, and nuts. Refrigerate until needed.

For the fish: Cut the fillets into 1 inch cubes. You should end up with 48 pieces. Place the fish in a plastic bag. Mix the garlic, oil, lime juice, and red pepper flakes in a bowl. Add to the fish, mix carefully, and refrigerate for 1 hour.

Preheat the broiler. Remove the fish pieces from the bag and pat dry. Cover a baking sheet with parchment paper. Add the fish pieces and broil for 2 to 3 minutes. Turn over and cook until the flesh starts to flake.

Place 2 fish pieces in the center of a romaine leaf and spoon over some chutney. Slightly fold over the leaf and serve immediately.

The cooked monkfish and chutney may be kept refrigerated separately up to 2 days.

SERVING SIZE: 1 filled Romaine leaf

PER SERVING: 117 Cal (53% from Fat, 36% from Protein, 12% from Carb); 11 g Protein; 7 g Tot Fat; 1 g Sat Fat; 4 g Mono Fat; 3 g Carb; 1 g Fiber; 2 g Sugar; 57 mg Calcium; 1 mg Iron; 29 mg Sodium; 15 mg Cholesterol

YIELD: 24 servings

Petites Tomates à la Morue
(CHERRY TOMATOES WITH COD FISH)

Place the salted cod fish in cold water. Refrigerate for 24 hours to desalt. If possible, change the water 3 or 4 times during the 24 hours.

Heat a nonstick pan with a thin layer of oil over medium heat. Add the fish and slightly brown. Turn over, reduce heat, and continue to cook until the flesh begins to flake. Remove the fish from the pan and set aside to cool. Once cold, shred the fish into small pieces.

Cut the tops of the tomatoes and set them aside for later use. With a melon baller empty the tomatoes. Be careful not to break their bottoms or sides. Turn the empty tomatoes upside down on a plate and set aside.

In a bowl mix the shallot, garlic, parsley, chives, scallions, lime juice, and 1 tablespoon olive oil. Add the pepper and a few drops of hot sauce. Add the cod fish and mix well. Stuff the tomatoes with the fish mixture and add the tomatoes tops. Refrigerate for 30 minutes before serving.

The cod mixture may be refrigerated up to 2 days.

1 pound salted cod fish
1 shallot, minced
1 garlic clove, minced
1 bunch fresh parsley, minced
1 bunch fresh chives, minced
2 ounces scallions, chopped thinly
    (about 5 scallions)
1 3/4 cup lime juice
1 tablespoon olive oil
24 cherry tomatoes
A few drops of hot sauce
Pepper

SERVING SIZE: 1 tomato

PER SERVING: 69 Cal (14% from Fat, 70% from Protein, 15% from Carb); 12 g Protein; 1 g Tot Fat; 0 g Sat Fat; 0 g Mono Fat; 3 g Carb; 0 g Fiber; 0 g Sugar; 35 mg Calcium; 1 mg Iron; 1329 mg Sodium; 29 mg Cholesterol

YIELD: 24 servings

Roulades de Saumon Fumé
(SMOKED SALMON ROLLS)

Cut the bell peppers in half. Remove seeds and ribs. Slice each half into 6 equal slices and set aside. This results in a total of 24 slices per color.

Remove the unusable ends from the scallions. Cut the scallions to the same size as the bell peppers and set aside.

Peel the kiwis. Cut each kiwi into 4 slices and set aside.

Heat 1 teaspoon of oil in a nonstick pan over high heat. Add the bell peppers and sauté for 2 to 3 minutes, mixing occasionally. Remove from the pan and set aside in a platter. Add 1 teaspoon of oil, the scallions, and sauté for 2 minutes. Remove from pan and set aside in a platter. Once cool, cut the scallions in half (lengthwise) and set aside in the platter.

In a bowl mix the cream cheese, chives, dill, shallot, and pepper. Add a little lemon juice to thin out.

Place one salmon fillet over a plastic wrap. Spread 1 teaspoon of flavored cream cheese over the fillet. Add 1 slice of the red bell pepper, one slice of the yellow bell pepper, and 1/2 scallion. Sprinkle with a little lemon juice and roll tightly. Top with 1 kiwi slice and set with a toothpick.

The salmon, cream cheese, and vegetables may be kept refrigerated separately up to 2 days.

24 slices smoked salmon (about 1 pound, 2 ounces smoked salmon)

8 tablespoons cream cheese

1 tablespoon fresh chives, minced

2 teaspoons fresh dill, minced

1 small shallot, minced

2 large red bell peppers

2 large yellow bell peppers

12 scallions

2 lemons

6 kiwis

2 teaspoons olive oil

Pepper to taste

24 wooden toothpicks

SERVING SIZE: 1 salmon roll

PER SERVING: 50 Cal (39% from Fat, 13% from Protein, 48% from Carb); 2 g Protein; 2 g Tot Fat; 1 g Sat Fat; 1 g Mono Fat; 7 g Carb; 2 g Fiber; 3 g Sugar; 25 mg Calcium; 0 mg Iron; 45 mg Sodium; 6 mg Cholesterol

YIELD: 24 servings

Spinach Boreks

Squeeze the spinach to remove as much water as possible. In a food processor combine the spinach, scallions, parsley, dill, garlic, cheeses, eggs, and nutmeg. Season to taste and refrigerate for 20 minutes.

Cut the phyllo dough to fit a 9 by 13-inch greased cake pan. Once you open the phyllo dough package, work as quickly as possible. Always keep the phyllo dough covered with plastic wrap and a damp towel to avoid dryness. First brush with oil the edges of one sheet and then the center. Repeat until you end up with a total of 10 sheets. Place the sheets on the bottom of the pan. Spread the filling evenly. Repeat the oiling process with the remaining 10 sheets. Place these sheets on top of the filling and press to set. Cover with plastic wrap and a damp cloth, and refrigerate for 20 minutes.

1 pound phyllo dough, thawed
3/4 cup grapeseed oil
10 ounces frozen spinach, thawed and chopped
1/4 cup scallions, chopped small
1/4 cup fresh parsley, minced
1 tablespoon fresh dill, minced
2 garlic cloves, minced
3/4 cup feta cheese, crumbled
1/4 cup Monterey Jack cheese, shredded
2 large eggs
1/2 teaspoon nutmeg
Salt and pepper to taste

Preheat the oven to 350 degrees F. Using a very sharp knife cut 1 1/2-inch squares into the dough. You should end up with 48 pieces. Bake for 45 minutes or until golden brown. Serve immediately.

The boreks may be refrigerated up to 2 days.

You may freeze cooked boreks up to 1 month. Reheat at 350 degrees F for 15 to 20 minutes.

SERVING SIZE: 1 borek

PER SERVING: 73 Cal (61% from Fat, 9% from Protein, 30% from Carb); 2 g Protein; 5 g Tot Fat; 1 g Sat Fat; 2 g Mono Fat; 5 g Carb; 0 g Fiber; 0 g Sugar; 29 mg Calcium; 1 mg Iron; 85 mg Sodium; 13 mg Cholesterol

YIELD: 48 servings

Carottes Glacées au Jus d'Orange
(ORANGE-GLAZED CARROTS)

Heat the oil in a saucepan over high heat. Add the onions, carrots, and brown slightly. Add the honey and barely enough orange juice to cover the vegetables (about 1 1/2 cups). Bring to boil and cook over medium heat until the liquid is almost completely evaporated. Add the chopped parsley and season to taste.

You may add flavoring, such as coriander seeds, if appropriate with the accompaniment.

The carrots may be refrigerated up to 5 days.

The carrots may be frozen up to 1 month.

1 tablespoon grapeseed oil

1 1/2 pounds baby carrots (about 6 cups baby carrots)

4 ounces sweet onions, diced (about 1 small sweet onion)

1 teaspoon orange blossom honey

1 1/2 cups orange juice

3 tablespoons fresh parsley, minced

Salt and pepper to taste

SERVING SIZE: 4 ounces

PER SERVING: 106 Cal (22% from Fat, 6% from Protein, 72% from Carb); 2 g Protein; 3 g Tot Fat; 0 g Sat Fat; 1 g Mono Fat; 20 g Carb; 4 g Fiber; 7 g Sugar; 50 mg Calcium; 1 mg Iron; 81 mg Sodium; 0 mg Cholesterol

YIELD: 6 servings

Cèpes à la Provençale
(PORCINI MUSHROOMS PROVENCE STYLE)

2 pounds Porcini mushrooms

2 tablespoons garlic cloves, minced

2 tablespoons fresh parsley, minced

1 teaspoon fresh thyme, minced

1 tablespoon fresh basil, minced

3 tablespoons olive oil

Salt and pepper to taste

Clean the mushrooms and pat dry. Slice the mushrooms and set aside.

Heat the oil in a large nonstick pan over medium heat. Add the garlic and cook for 15 seconds. Add the mushrooms, thyme, and sauté for 2 to 3 minutes. Add the parsley, basil, and season to taste. Continue to cook for 2 minutes and serve immediately.

The mushrooms may be refrigerated up to 2 days, though they taste better when cooked and served immediately.

SERVING SIZE: 1/4 recipe

PER SERVING: 150 Cal (59% from Fat, 18% from Protein, 23% from Carb); 8 g Protein; 11 g Tot Fat; 1 g Sat Fat; 8 g Mono Fat; 10 g Carb; 3 g Fiber; 4 g Sugar; 19 mg Calcium; 2 mg Iron; 18 mg Sodium; 0 mg Cholesterol

YIELD: 4 servings

Couscous aux Petits Légumes
(Couscous with Vegetables)

Heat the oil in a nonstick pan over high heat. Add the onions and sauté until translucent. Add the garlic, carrots, celery, bell peppers, and cook for 3 minutes over medium heat. Add the lemon zest, lemon juice, parsley, almonds, and sauté for 1 minute. Season to taste and add 1 1/4 cups water. Bring to boil and mix in the couscous. Cover and removed from heat. Let stand for 5 minutes. Taste, adjust seasonings, and serve immediately.

The water may be replaced with stock (low-fat and low-sodium).

The couscous may be refrigerated up to 5 days.

The couscous may be frozen up to 1 month.

1 teaspoon olive oil

1 tablespoon garlic cloves, minced

4 ounces onions, diced small (about 1 small onion)

2 ounces carrots, diced small (about 1 small carrot)

2 ounces celery, diced small (about 1 large celery stalk)

2 ounces red bell peppers, diced small (about 1/2 medium red bell pepper)

1 cup uncooked wheat couscous

1 teaspoon lemon zest

2 tablespoons lemon juice

1/4 cup fresh parsley, minced

2 tablespoons almonds, chopped

Salt and pepper to taste

Serving Size: about 3/4 cup couscous or 1/4 recipe

Per Serving: 220 Cal (13% from Fat, 13% from Protein, 75% from Carb); 7 g Protein; 3 g Tot Fat; 0 g Sat Fat; 2 g Mono Fat; 41 g Carb; 4 g Fiber; 3 g Sugar; 45 mg Calcium; 1 mg Iron; 29 mg Sodium; 0 mg Cholesterol

Yield: 4 servings

Epinards aux Raisins de Corinth
(SPINACH WITH PINE NUTS AND RAISINS)

Heat the oil in a nonstick pan over medium heat. Add the raisins, and pine nuts, and sauté for 1 minute. Add the spinach and sauté very briefly. Season to taste and serve immediately. The spinach should be barely cooked to avoid turning to mush.

The spinach may be refrigerated up to 2 days.

Freezing is not recommended.

2 tablespoons grapeseed oil

2 pounds fresh spinach, washed and pat dry

2 ounces plump raisins (a little more than 1/3 cup)

1 tablespoon pine nuts

Salt and pepper to taste

SERVING SIZE: 1/4 recipe

PER SERVING: 187 Cal (42% from Fat, 18% from Protein, 40% from Carb); 10 g Protein; 10 g Tot Fat; 2 g Sat Fat; 4 g Mono Fat; 21 g Carb; 8 g Fiber; 10 g Sugar; 359 mg Calcium; 5 mg Iron; 169 mg Sodium; 0 mg Cholesterol

YIELD: 4 servings

Haricots Verts aux Tomates
(Green Beans with Tomatoes)

Bring to boil enough water to cover the green beans. Add 1 teaspoon of salt. Add the green beans and bring to a boil. Reduce heat and simmer until tender. Drain and set aside.

1 1/2 tablespoons olive oil
1 pound green beans, ends trimmed
1 cup cherry tomatoes
1/2 cup pearl onions, peeled and halved
2 garlic cloves, minced
2 pinches fresh thyme, minced
2 tablespoons fresh basil, minced
1 tablespoon fresh parsley, minced
Salt and pepper to taste

Heat 1 tablespoon of oil in a nonstick pan over medium heat. Add the pearl onions and sauté until golden brown. Add the garlic and cook for 1 minute. Add the green beans, tomatoes, herbs, and cook until the vegetables are warm. Blend in the remaining oil, season to taste, and serve immediately.

The green beans and tomatoes may be refrigerated up to 2 days.

Freezing is not recommended.

Serving Size: 1/4 recipe

Per Serving: 100 Cal (44% from Fat, 10% from Protein, 46% from Carb); 3 g Protein; 5 g Tot Fat; 1 g Sat Fat; 4 g Mono Fat; 13 g Carb; 5 g Fiber; 3 g Sugar; 54 mg Calcium; 2 mg Iron; 8 mg Sodium; 0 mg Cholesterol

Yield: 4 servings

Légumes à la Vapeur
(STEAMED VEGETABLES)

Steaming is a very fast cooking process, so pay attention because your vegetables can be overcooked very quickly. Cut the vegetables the same size for even cooking.

Mix the lemon juice, herbs, and set aside.

Preheat a steamer. When the water is boiling, add the carrots and cauliflower florets in even layers to ensure uniform cooking. Cook covered for 4 minutes. Add the broccoli florets, cover, and cook for 1 to 2 minutes. Transfer the vegetables to a serving bowl. Mix in the lemon juice mixture, season to taste, and serve immediately.

The vegetables may be refrigerated up to 5 days.

The vegetables may be frozen up to 1 month.

8 ounces baby carrots (about 2 cups baby carrots)
8 ounces broccoli florets (about 1 medium head broccoli florets)
8 ounces cauliflower florets (about 1/2 small head cauliflower florets)
1 tablespoon fresh salad herbs
1 lemon, juiced
Salt and pepper to taste

SERVING SIZE: 6 ounces

PER SERVING: 56 Cal (8% from Fat, 19% from Protein, 73% from Carb); 3 g Protein; 1 g Tot Fat; 0 g Sat Fat; 0 g Mono Fat; 13 g Carb; 6 g Fiber; 4 g Sugar; 76 mg Calcium; 1 mg Iron; 62 mg Sodium; 0 mg Cholesterol

YIELD: 4 servings

Légumes Grillés à la Vinaigrette d'Anchois
(GRILLED VEGETABLES WITH ANCHOVY VINAIGRETTE)

For the marinade: Using a food processor purée the garlic, capers, and anchovy fillets. Add the vinegar, olive oil, lemon juice, parsley, dill, and mix well.

For the vegetables: Cut the vegetables to the same size for even cooking. Parboil the carrots for 2 minutes and place immediately in ice-cold water. Parboil the cauliflower for 1 minute and place immediately in ice-cold water. Pat dry the vegetables.

Place all the vegetables in a plastic bag, add marinade, mix well, and refrigerate for a minimum of 4 hours.

Preheat the oven to 450 degrees F. Transfer the vegetables and marinade to a baking pan. Sprinkle with some pepper to taste. Bake for 20 to 25 minutes or until desired doneness. Sprinkle with salt and serve immediately.

FOR THE VEGETABLES:

8 ounces broccoli florets (about 1 medium head broccoli florets)

8 ounces carrots (about 2 large carrots)

8 ounces cauliflower florets (about 1/2 small head cauliflower florets)

6 ounces onions (about 1 medium onion)

6 ounces yellow zucchini (about 1 large yellow zucchini)

6 ounces red bell peppers (about 1 large red bell pepper)

Salt and pepper to taste

FOR THE MARINADE:

1 tablespoon garlic cloves, minced

1 tablespoon capers

1 ounce anchovy fillets

2 tablespoons white wine vinegar

4 tablespoons olive oil

2 tablespoons lemon juice

1/4 cup fresh parsley, chopped

1 dill branch, minced

These cooked vegetables are also great cold in a salad.

The vegetables may be refrigerated up to 5 days.

The vegetables may be frozen up to 1 month.

SERVING SIZE: 6 ounces vegetables

PER SERVING: 113 Cal (55% from Fat, 11% from Protein, 34% from Carb); 3 g Protein; 7 g Tot Fat; 1 g Sat Fat; 5 g Mono Fat; 10 g Carb; 3 g Fiber; 4 g Sugar; 52 mg Calcium; 1 mg Iron; 199 mg Sodium; 3 mg Cholesterol

YIELD: 8 servings

Tagine de Blette
(Swiss Chard Tagine)

Wash the Swiss chard and blanch in simmering salted water for 2 minutes. Strain and press out excess water. Let cool and chop.

Heat the oil in a nonstick pan over high heat. Add the onions, garlic, and sauté for 2 minutes. Add the Swiss chard and cook for 5 minutes or until tender. Sprinkle with salt, pepper, and paprika to taste. Mix well and serve immediately.

The tagine may be refrigerated up to 5 days.

Not recommended for freezing.

2 pounds Swiss chard

4 ounces onions, diced (about 1 small onion)

3 tablespoons olive oil

1 tablespoon garlic cloves, minced

Salt, pepper, and paprika, to taste

Serving Size: 1/4 recipe

Per Serving: 148 Cal (59% from Fat, 11% from Protein, 30% from Carb); 4 g Protein; 11 g Tot Fat; 1 g Sat Fat; 8 g Mono Fat; 12 g Carb; 4 g Fiber; 4 g Sugar; 126 mg Calcium; 4 mg Iron; 485 mg Sodium; 0 mg Cholesterol

Yield: 4 servings

Tomates à la Provençale
(TOMATOES PROVENCE STYLE)

Preheat the oven to 375 degrees F.

Cut the tomatoes in half. Sprinkle 1/4 teaspoon olive oil over each half. Add some garlic and season to taste. Sprinkle some basil and 1 teaspoon bread crumbs over each half. Place in a baking dish, sprinkle the remaining oil over the bread crumbs, and bake for 20 to 25 minutes. Serve immediately.

The tomatoes may be refrigerated up to 2 days.

Not recommended for freezing.

4 large tomatoes

2 tablespoons olive oil

2 tablespoons garlic cloves, minced

1 bunch of fresh basil leaves, minced

1/4 cup bread crumbs

Salt and pepper to taste

SERVING SIZE: 1 tomato

PER SERVING: 130 Cal (49% from Fat, 8% from Protein, 43% from Carb); 3 g Protein; 8 g Tot Fat; 1 g Sat Fat; 5 g Mono Fat; 15 g Carb; 2 g Fiber; 0 g Sugar; 25 mg Calcium; 1 mg Iron; 215 mg Sodium; 0 mg Cholesterol

YIELD: 4 servings

Gratin de Légumes au Thym
(VEGETABLES GRATIN WITH THYME)

Cut the vegetables the same size for even cooking.

In a bowl mix the garlic, lemon juice, stock, thyme, parsley, a pinch of salt, and a pinch of pepper. Mix in the remaining vegetables (except sweet potatoes) and set aside for at least an hour.

Preheat the oven to 425 degrees F. Place the sweet potatoes in a roasting pan. Mix in half of the olive oil, sprinkle with pepper, and bake for 20 minutes. Sprinkle the remaining oil over the potatoes. Add the prepared vegetables with the marinade and continue to bake for 20 minutes. Sprinkle with the cheese, brown under the broiler, and serve immediately.

The gratin may be refrigerated up to 5 days.

The gratin may be frozen up to 1 month.

Add the cheese after reheating.

SERVING SIZE: 1/8 recipe

PER SERVING: 197 Cal (40% from Fat, 13% from Protein, 47% from Carb); 7 g Protein; 9 g Tot Fat; 2 g Sat Fat; 6 g Mono Fat; 25 g Carb; 4 g Fiber; 9 g Sugar; 147 mg Calcium; 2 mg Iron; 145 mg Sodium; 6 mg Cholesterol

YIELD: 8 servings

12 ounces yellow squash, chopped large (about 2 large yellow squash)

12 ounces red bell peppers, seeded, ribs removed, and chopped large (about 2 large red bell peppers)

12 ounces broccoli florets (about 1 medium head plus 1 small head broccoli florets)

12 ounces zucchini, chopped large (about 2 large zucchini)

1 pound onions, quartered (about 2 large onions)

1 pound sweet potatoes, chopped large (about 3 medium sweet potatoes)

4 large garlic cloves, minced

2 tablespoons lemon juice

2 tablespoons vegetable stock (low-sodium)

4 tablespoons olive oil

2 fresh thyme branches, minced

3 tablespoons fresh parsley, minced

2 ounces Parmesan cheese, grated

Salt and pepper to taste

Poivrons Farcis
(STUFFED BELL PEPPERS)

4 large red bell peppers

1 tablespoon olive oil

4 ounces onions, diced (about 1 small onion)

2 garlic cloves, minced

5 ounces tomatoes (about 1 large tomato)

10 ounces cooked brown rice

5 ounces vegetable stock (low-sodium)

3 tablespoons fresh parsley, minced

2 pinches dried Italian herbs, minced

8 ounces tomato sauce

Salt and pepper to taste

Make a small X incision on the top and bottom of the tomatoes. Blanch the tomatoes for 20 seconds. Place in ice-cold water to stop the cooking process. Peel, seed, and dice the tomatoes.

Wash the bell peppers and cut off their tops. Remove ribs and seeds. Parboil the bell peppers for 2 minutes. Remove the bell peppers from the pan and invert to drain over paper towels.

Heat the oil in a nonstick pan over high heat. Add the onions and sauté until translucent. Add the garlic, rice, tomatoes, parsley, Italian herbs, 3 ounces stock, and bring to a boil. Season to taste and remove from heat. Cool down completely before filling the bell peppers with this mixture. Finish by replacing their tops.

Preheat the oven to 350 degrees F. Place the stuffed bell peppers in a greased pan. Add the remaining stock to the pan and bake for 25 to 30 minutes.

Heat the tomato sauce and serve immediately with the stuffed bell peppers.

The stuffed bell peppers may be refrigerated up to 5 days.

The stuffed bell peppers may be frozen up to 1 month. Be aware that the bell peppers will be a little mushy when reheated.

SERVING SIZE: 1 stuffed bell pepper

PER SERVING: 200 Cal (21% from Fat, 10% from Protein, 70% from Carb); 5 g Protein; 5 g Tot Fat; 1 g Sat Fat; 3 g Mono Fat; 37 g Carb; 6 g Fiber; 12 g Sugar; 47 mg Calcium; 2 mg Iron; 328 mg Sodium; 0 mg Cholesterol

YIELD: 4 servings

Aubergine Farcie
(STUFFED EGGPLANT)

1 pound eggplant (about 2 medium eggplants)

1 egg

6 ounces onions, diced (about 1 medium onion)

2 tablespoons garlic cloves, minced

3 tablespoons olive oil

1/2 cup Italian bread crumbs

4 basil leaves, minced

1/4 cup fresh parsley, minced

Salt and pepper to taste

Place the egg in a saucepan and cover with water. Bring to boil over medium heat and then cook for 10 minutes. Strain and cool in cold water. Peel the egg and mash with a fork in a bowl.

Preheat the oven to 425 degrees F. Cut the eggplants in half and remove the flesh without damaging the skin. Make very small incisions on the rim tops; this will prevent breakage during cooking. Place the eggplant halves in a small greased baking pan and brush them with olive oil. In a food processor purée the eggplant flesh and mashed egg.

Heat 1 teaspoon olive oil in a nonstick pan over medium heat. Add the onions, garlic, and sauté for 2 minutes. Add the eggplant mixture, herbs, and cook for 2 minutes. Season to taste and fill the eggplant cavities with this mixture. Spread the bread crumbs over the eggplant halves and sprinkle with a little olive oil. Bake for 30 to 35 minutes.

The eggplant may be refrigerated up to 2 days.

Not recommended for freezing.

SERVING SIZE: 1/2 eggplant

PER SERVING: 219 Cal (49% from Fat, 10% from Protein, 41% from Carb); 6 g Protein; 12 g Tot Fat; 2 g Sat Fat; 8 g Mono Fat; 23 g Carb; 5 g Fiber; 5 g Sugar; 57 mg Calcium; 1 mg Iron; 425 mg Sodium; 61 mg Cholesterol

YIELD: 4 servings

Broccoli à la Vinaigrette de Pistache
(BROCCOLI WITH PISTACHIO VINAIGRETTE)

In a bowl mix the mustard, shallot, garlic, oil, lemon juice, parsley, and season to taste.

Preheat a steamer. Add the broccoli and cook for 2 to 3 minutes or until desired doneness. Heat the vinaigrette, toss with the warm broccoli, and serve immediately.

You may substitute 2 tablespoons balsamic vinegar for the lemon juice.

The broccoli (without the vinaigrette) may be refrigerated up to 5 days.

The broccoli (without the vinaigrette) may be frozen up to 1 month.

Add the vinaigrette after reheating.

1 1/2 pounds broccoli florets (about 2 1/2 large heads broccoli florets)

1 teaspoon Dijon mustard

1 tablespoon shallots, minced

1 teaspoon garlic cloves, minced

4 tablespoons pistachio oil

3 tablespoons lemon juice

1 tablespoon fresh parsley, minced

Salt and pepper to taste

SERVING SIZE: 6 ounces

PER SERVING: 175 Cal (67% from Fat, 11% from Protein, 22% from Carb); 5 g Protein; 14 g Tot Fat; 1 g Sat Fat; 3 g Mono Fat; 11 g Carb; 0 g Fiber; 0 g Sugar; 87 mg Calcium; 2 mg Iron; 62 mg Sodium; 0 mg Cholesterol

YIELD: 4 servings

Légumes Marinés au Citron
(MARINATED VEGETABLES WITH LEMON)

For the marinade: Remove zest from the lemon, mince, and place in a bowl. Juice the lemon and add to the bowl. Blend in the remaining marinade ingredients and set aside.

For the vegetables: Cut the vegetables the same size for even cooking. Parboil the carrots for 2 minutes and place immediately in ice-cold water.

Place all the vegetables in a plastic bag, add the marinade, mix well, and refrigerate for a minimum of 4 hours.

Preheat the oven to 450 F. Transfer the vegetables and marinade to a baking pan. Sprinkle some pepper to taste. Bake for 20 to 25 minutes or until desired doneness. Sprinkle with salt and serve immediately.

The vegetables may be refrigerated up to 5 days.

The vegetables may be frozen up to 1 month.

FOR THE VEGETABLES:
8 ounces onions (about 1 large onion)
8 ounces carrots (about 2 large carrots)
8 ounces asparagus (about 8 asparagus)
8 ounces broccoli florets (about 1 medium head broccoli florets)

FOR THE MARINADE:
1 lemon
1 tablespoon garlic cloves, minced
1 branch fresh thyme, minced
1 teaspoon honey
1 tablespoon rice vinegar
3 tablespoons olive oil
1 teaspoon dry parsley
Salt and pepper to taste

SERVING SIZE: 6 ounces

PER SERVING: 178 Cal (48% from Fat, 9% from Protein, 43% from Carb); 4 g Protein; 11 g Tot Fat; 1 g Sat Fat; 8 g Mono Fat; 22 g Carb; 5 g Fiber; 8 g Sugar; 93 mg Calcium; 2 mg Iron; 59 mg Sodium; 0 mg Cholesterol

YIELD: 4 servings

Pâtes aux Artichauds et Tomates Confites
(PASTA WITH SUN-DRIED TOMATOES AND ARTICHOKE)

Fill a stockpot 3/4 full with water, add 1 teaspoon canola oil, and bring to boil over high heat. Add the penne and cook until al dente. Drain and transfer to a bowl. Mix in one tablespoon of olive oil.

Heat 2 tablespoons olive oil in a large nonstick pan over high heat. Add the onions and sauté until translucent. Add the artichokes, squash, thyme, garlic, lemon juice, and sauté for 3 minutes. Add the mushrooms, sun-dried tomatoes, peas, basil, parsley, and season to taste. Cook for 3 minutes. Add the pasta, mix well, and continue to cook until all the ingredients are warm. Transfer to a pasta dish, sprinkle with Parmesan cheese, and serve immediately.

1 pound artichoke hearts (frozen)
1 teaspoon canola oil
3 tablespoons olive oil
6 ounces red onions, julienned (about 1 medium red onion)
6 ounces yellow squash, julienned (about 1 large yellow squash)
1/2 cup frozen peas
1/2 cup sun-dried tomatoes, julienned
4 ounces crimini mushrooms, sliced
1 tablespoon fresh thyme, minced
1/2 cup fresh basil, chopped
3 tablespoons garlic cloves, minced
2 tablespoons lemon juice
4 tablespoons Parmesan cheese
1 cup whole grain penne
2 tablespoons fresh parsley, minced
Salt and pepper to taste

If using a jar of sun-dried tomatoes, substitute 1 tablespoon of their oil for the 1 tablespoon of oil referred to when mixing with the pasta.

The dish may be refrigerated up to 5 days.

The dish may be frozen separately up to 1 month.

SERVING SIZE: 1/4 recipe

PER SERVING: 361 Cal (38% from Fat, 12% from Protein, 49% from Carb); 12 g Protein; 16 g Tot Fat; 3 g Sat Fat; 10 g Mono Fat; 48 g Carb; 12 g Fiber; 5 g Sugar; 152 mg Calcium; 3 mg Iron; 264 mg Sodium; 6 mg Cholesterol

YIELD: 4 servings

Purée de Pommes de Terre et Navets
(POTATO PARSNIP PURÉE)

Peel and quarter the potatoes and parsnips. Place them in a deep pan and add enough cold water to cover them. Add the garlic cloves, 1/4 teaspoon salt, and bring to boil over high heat. Cook until tender, about 20 to 25 minutes. Pass through a sieve, keeping some of the cooking liquid, and purée with a potato masher. Add milk, olive oil, and mix quickly. If too thick, add a little cooking liquid to get to the right consistency. Mix in the parsley, chives, and season to taste. Serve immediately.

3 pounds white potatoes (about 8 medium potatoes)
3 large garlic cloves, peeled
6 ounces parsnips (about 1 large parsnip)
1/2 cup milk
1 tablespoon fresh parsley, minced
1 tablespoon fresh chives, minced
1 tablespoon olive oil
Salt and pepper to taste

The purée may be refrigerated up to 5 days.

The purée may be frozen up to 1 month.

Add a little milk before reheating to avoid dryness.

SERVING SIZE: 1/8 recipe

PER SERVING: 158 Cal (12% from Fat, 9% from Protein, 79% from Carb); 4 g Protein; 2 g Tot Fat; 0 g Sat Fat; 1 g Mono Fat; 32 g Carb; 5 g Fiber; 4 g Sugar; 44 mg Calcium; 1 mg Iron; 20 mg Sodium; 1 mg Cholesterol

YIELD: 8 servings

Ragoût d'Haricots
(WHITE BEAN STEW)

Place the beans in a large stockpot and add enough water to cover them. Bring to a boil over high heat. Remove from heat and let stand covered for 30 minutes. Drain the beans and rinse under cold water.

Heat the oil in a large pan over high heat. Add the onions, carrots, celery, garlic, and sauté for 2 minutes. Mix in the flour. Add the beans, bouquet garni, and 4 cups stock. If the beans are not covered, add enough water to do so. Bring to boil, reduce heat, and simmer covered for 1 to 1 1/2 hours or until tender. Add the tomato purée and bring to a boil. Add parsley and season to taste. If the mixture is too thin, remove some beans, mash them, and add to them back to the stew. Serve immediately.

1 teaspoon olive oil
2 pounds dried white beans
6 ounces onions, diced (about 1 medium onion)
3 ounces carrots, diced (about 1 medium carrot)
3 ounces celery stalks, diced (about 2 medium celery stalks)
2 tablespoons garlic cloves, minced
15 ounces canned tomato purée
1 tablespoon flour
2 tablespoons fresh parsley, minced
1 bouquet garni
4 cups chicken stock (low-fat and low-sodium)
Salt and pepper to taste

Substitute chicken stock with vegetable stock.

The stew may be refrigerated up to 5 days.

The stew may be frozen up to 1 month.

SERVING SIZE: 1/8 recipe

PER SERVING: 461 Cal (5% from Fat, 24% from Protein, 71% from Carb); 29 g Protein; 3 g Tot Fat; 1 g Sat Fat; 1 g Mono Fat; 84 g Carb; 19 g Fiber; 8 g Sugar; 310 mg Calcium; 14 mg Iron; 461 mg Sodium; 1 mg Cholesterol

YIELD: 8 servings

Ratatouille

Make a small X incision on the top and bottom of the tomatoes. Blanch the tomatoes for 20 seconds. Place in ice-cold water to stop the cooking process. Peel, seed, and dice the tomatoes.

Heat the oil in a large deep pan over high heat. Add the onions, bell peppers, garlic, and sauté for 2 to 3 minutes. Add the eggplant, zucchini, and orange juice. Cover, reduce heat, and cook for 15 minutes. Add the tomatoes, bay leaf, herbs de Provence, and continue to cook uncovered over low heat for 25 to 30 minutes. If necessary, cook a little longer until the consistency is a little thick. Add the parsley and basil. Season to taste and serve immediately.

The ratatouille may be refrigerated up to 5 days.

The ratatouille may be frozen up to 1 month.

4 tablespoons olive oil
1 pound zucchini, diced (about 3 large zucchinis)
1 pound eggplant, peeled and diced (about 2 medium eggplants)
1 pound onions, thinly sliced (about 2 large onions)
12 ounces red bell peppers, thinly sliced (about 2 large red bell peppers)
12 ounces yellow bell peppers, thinly sliced (about 2 large yellow bell peppers)
2 tablespoons garlic cloves, minced
2 pounds tomatoes (about 6 large tomatoes)
4 ounces orange juice
1/4 cup fresh parsley, minced
10 fresh basil leaves, minced
1 bay leaf
1 teaspoon herbs de Provence
Salt and pepper to taste

SERVING SIZE: 1/8 recipe

PER SERVING: 163 Cal (38% from Fat, 9% from Protein, 53% from Carb); 4 g Protein; 8 g Tot Fat; 1 g Sat Fat; 5 g Mono Fat; 24 g Carb; 6 g Fiber; 7 g Sugar; 48 mg Calcium; 2 mg Iron; 22 mg Sodium; 0 mg Cholesterol

YIELD: 8 servings

Risotto aux Olives
(Risotto with Olives)

Make a small X incision on the top and bottom of the tomatoes. Blanch the tomatoes for 20 seconds. Place in ice-cold water to stop the cooking process. Peel, seed, and dice the tomatoes.

Heat the oil in a pan over high heat. Add the onions and sauté until translucent. Add the garlic, rice, and stir for 1 minute. Add the wine, thyme, saffron, and cook until the liquid is evaporated over medium heat. Add half of the stock and simmer uncovered. Once the liquid is absorbed, add the remaining stock, olives, and continue to simmer uncovered. Once the stock is almost absorbed, add the tomatoes, Parmesan cheese, cream, herbs, and season to taste. Remove from heat and cover for 2 minutes before serving.

The risotto may be refrigerated up to 5 days.

The risotto may be frozen up to 1 month.

When reheating, add a little stock.

12 ounces Arborio rice

4 cups chicken stock (low-fat and low-sodium)

4 ounces onions, diced (about 1 small onion, diced)

1 tablespoon garlic cloves, minced

1 tablespoon olive oil

1 pound tomatoes (about 3 large tomatoes)

1/4 cup Parmesan cheese, grated

4 ounces Chardonnay wine

1/8 cup cream, heated

1/4 cup green olives, pitted

1 teaspoon dried thyme, minced

3 sprigs saffron

3 tablespoons fresh salad herbs, minced

Salt and pepper to taste

Serving Size: 1/8 recipe

Per Serving: 137 Cal (31% from Fat, 15% from Protein, 55% from Carb); 5 g Protein; 4 g Tot Fat; 2 g Sat Fat; 2 g Mono Fat; 18 g Carb; 1 g Fiber; 1 g Sugar; 63 mg Calcium; 2 mg Iron; 370 mg Sodium; 6 mg Cholesterol

Yield: 8 servings

Riz aux Lentilles
(RICE WITH LENTILS)

Place the lentils in a pan and cover with water. Bring to boil over high heat and simmer for 10 minutes. Strain and set aside.

Heat the oil in a large pan over high heat. Add the onions and sauté until translucent. Add the garlic, lentils, seasonings, and 6 cups water. Bring to a boil, reduce heat, cover, and simmer for 10 minutes. Add the rice and bring to a boil. Reduce heat, cover, and cook for 20 minutes or until tender. Adjust seasonings and remove from heat. Set aside covered for 5 minutes before serving.

The rice may be refrigerated up to 5 days.

The rice may be frozen up to 1 month.

8 ounces raw long-grain rice, rinsed (about 1 1/3 cup raw long-grain rice)

10 ounces lentils, rinsed (about 2 1/2 cups lentils)

1 pound onions, diced (about 2 large onions)

2 teaspoons garlic cloves, minced

2 teaspoons olive oil

1 teaspoon ground cumin

1 teaspoon ground coriander

1 teaspoon paprika

2 tablespoons fresh parsley

Salt and pepper to taste

SERVING SIZE: 1/8 recipe

PER SERVING: 184 Cal (11% from Fat, 13% from Protein, 76% from Carb); 6 g Protein; 2 g Tot Fat; 0 g Sat Fat; 1 g Mono Fat; 36 g Carb; 5 g Fiber; 3 g Sugar; 36 mg Calcium; 2 mg Iron; 7 mg Sodium; 0 mg Cholesterol

YIELD: 8 servings

Riz Sauvage aux Petits Légumes
(WILD RICE WITH VEGETABLES)

8 ounces raw wild rice (about 1 1/3 cup raw wild rice)

Rinse the rice well and drain. Heat the oil in a deep pan over high heat. Add the vegetables and sauté for 2 minutes. Add the rice and sauté for a minute. Add the stock, parsley, and bring to a boil. Cover, reduce heat, and cook until tender (approximately 45 minutes, but it may depend of the type of rice you use. For best result, see package instructions). Adjust seasonings and remove from heat. If necessary, strain and serve immediately.

You may add fresh herbs based on the accompaniment flavor.

This rice may be refrigerated for 5 days.

This rice may be frozen for 1 month.

2 teaspoons olive oil

12 ounces onions, diced small (about 2 medium onions)

6 ounces carrots, diced small (about 2 medium carrots)

6 ounces celery, diced small (about 3 large celery stalks)

1 garlic clove, minced

4 cups vegetable stock

2 tablespoons fresh parsley, minced

Salt and pepper to taste

SERVING SIZE: 1/8 recipe

PER SERVING: 173 Cal (12% from Fat, 9% from Protein, 78% from Carb); 4 g Protein; 2 g Tot Fat; 1 g Sat Fat; 1 g Mono Fat; 35 g Carb; 3 g Fiber; 5 g Sugar; 59 mg Calcium; 1 mg Iron; 101 mg Sodium; 0 mg Cholesterol

YIELD: 8 servings

CHAPTER

6

Desserts

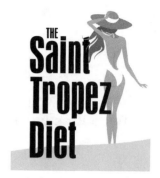

Salade de Fruits à la Menthe
(FRUIT SALAD WITH MINT)

Boil 3/4 cup of water. Add the lemon juice, tea sachet, honey, and infuse until desired strength. Remove sachet and cool completely.

Mix all the fruit in a large bowl. Add the cold tea and refrigerate for 30 minutes, mixing every 10 minutes. Mix in the fresh mint and serve immediately.

The salad may be refrigerated up to 2 days.

SERVING SIZE: 1/4 recipe

PER SERVING: 165 Cal (16% from Fat, 6% from Protein, 79% from Carb); 2 g Protein; 3 g Tot Fat; 1 g Sat Fat; 1 g Mono Fat; 34 g Carb; 5 g Fiber; 13 g Sugar; 31 mg Calcium; 1 mg Iron; 238 mg Sodium; 0 mg Cholesterol

YIELD: 4 servings

1 small banana, sliced
3 ounces strawberries, halved
3 ounces blueberries
3 ounces raspberries
1 small apple, cubed
2 large plums, quartered
1 mint tea sachet
1 tablespoon honey
1 tablespoon lemon juice
2 tablespoons fresh mint leaves, chopped

Soupe de Melon
(MELON SOUP)

Cut the cantaloupes in half. Remove seeds. Spoon out the flesh and place in a blender. Add the honey, mint, and lemon juice. Purée and refrigerate. Serve cold.

The soup may be refrigerated up to 2 days.

2 cantaloupes (or 4 cups net weight)

2 tablespoons honey (warmed in the microwave, about 10 seconds on high)

4 mint leaves

1 lemon, juiced

SERVING SIZE: 1 cup

PER SERVING: 98 Cal (3% from Fat, 6% from Protein, 90% from Carb); 2 g Protein; 0 g Tot Fat; 0 g Sat Fat; 0 g Mono Fat; 26 g Carb; 3 g Fiber; 23 g Sugar; 33 mg Calcium; 1 mg Iron; 30 mg Sodium; 0 mg Cholesterol

YIELD: 4 servings

Pêches Fourrées
(Stuffed Peaches)

Preheat the oven to 375 degrees F.

Cut the peaches in half and remove pits. Scoop out a little bit of the flesh from the center. Place the scooped flesh into a bowl and chop small. Crush the cookies and add to the bowl. Mix in the orange peel, honey, egg white, and almonds. Spoon the mixture equally into the peach halves. Top with a dash of butter. Place the stuffed peaches in the baking pan, add the wine, water, and bake for 25 to 30 minutes. Serve immediately.

4 peaches, washed and pat dry
4 to 5 Amoretti cookies
1 teaspoon orange peel, minced
1 tablespoon honey
1 large egg white
2 tablespoons blanched almonds, chopped
4 ounces white Muscat
2 ounces water
2 teaspoons butter

Serving Size: 1 peach

Per Serving: 191 Cal (27% from Fat, 8% from Protein, 65% from Carb); 4 g Protein; 5 g Tot Fat; 1 g Sat Fat; 2 g Mono Fat; 28 g Carb; 2 g Fiber; 16 g Sugar; 21 mg Calcium; 0 mg Iron; 19 mg Sodium; 5 mg Cholesterol

Yield: 4 servings

Compote de Figues au Yaourt
(FIGS COMPOTE WITH YOGURT)

2 cups figs

2 cups fresh orange juice

6 tablespoons orange blossom honey

1 large lemon peel, minced

1 large orange peel, minced

2 fresh rosemary branches

1 pound low-fat yogurt

2 ounces walnuts, chopped

Cut the figs in half lengthwise. In a saucepan combine the orange juice, peels, and rosemary. Bring to a boil over medium heat and simmer for 5 minutes. Remove rosemary, add the figs, honey, cover, and simmer for 15 minutes. Remove cover, mix crushing the figs a little bit, and thicken for 4 to 5 minutes. Remove from heat and cool down for 2 minutes. Strain, pressing hard to release as much as possible of the figs flesh. Discard skins. Refrigerate at least for 2 hours before serving.

Prepare 8 dessert dishes. Place 2 ounces of yogurt in each and top with the fig compote. Sprinkle with the walnuts and serve immediately.

You can use dried figs, though the flavor will not be as good. To rehydrate them, cover the figs with water overnight.

The compote may be kept refrigerated 5 days.

SERVING SIZE: 1/8 recipe

PER SERVING: 251 Cal (20% from Fat, 9% from Protein, 72% from Carb); 6 g Protein; 6 g Tot Fat; 1 g Sat Fat; 1 g Mono Fat; 48 g Carb; 4 g Fiber; 40 g Sugar; 179 mg Calcium; 1 mg Iron; 45 mg Sodium; 3 mg Cholesterol

YIELD: 8 servings

Fraises au Vin Rouge Poivré
(STRAWBERRIES WITH SPICY RED WINE)

In a saucepan combine the red wine, honey, vanilla, peels, and peppercorns. Bring to a boil over high heat. Continue to boil until the wine is reduced by half. Remove from heat and strain.

Place the strawberries in a bowl and pour over the hot wine. Mix well and let cool. Refrigerate at least for two hours. Serve cold.

The dessert may be refrigerated up to 2 days.

1 pound strawberries

1 cup red wine (Chianti, Beaujolais, or Berg- erac)

3 tablespoons honey

1 teaspoon vanilla extract

1 orange peel

1 lemon peel

4 to 6 teaspoons black peppercorns, crushed

SERVING SIZE: 1/4 recipe

PER SERVING: 144 Cal (4% from Fat, 5% from Protein, 91% from Carb); 2 g Protein; 1 g Tot Fat; 0 g Sat Fat; 0 g Mono Fat; 26 g Carb; 4 g Fiber; 19 g Sugar; 47 mg Calcium; 2 mg Iron; 7 mg Sodium; 0 mg Cholesterol

YIELD: 4 servings

The Apostolos Crêpes

Place the flour in a bowl. Blend in the eggs, honey, vanilla, salt, and 2 tablespoons oil. Slowly whisk in the milk. Let the batter rest for 30 minutes. Before use, add a little water to thin out the batter.

Heat a nonstick pan or crêpe pan over medium heat. Soak a small piece of paper towel with 1 teaspoon grapeseed oil and swirl quickly over the pan. Add enough batter and swirl to cover the entire bottom. Cook until golden brown and turn over. Cook until slightly golden brown. Add filling or remove from pan and set aside for later use.

1 cup flour

2 extra-large eggs

1 tablespoon honey

2 tablespoons vanilla extract

Pinch salt

2 tablespoons plus 1 teaspoon grapeseed oil

1 cup milk

You can make a batch of crêpes and refrigerate them for up to 5 days. Place wax paper between each crêpe, and then wrap the whole batch tightly in foil. To reheat, preheat a medium skillet over medium heat. When warm, place a crêpe in the skillet and heat for a few seconds on each side until hot to the touch. Freezing is not really recommended for the types of fillings we've included.

SERVING SIZE: 1 crêpe

PER SERVING: 114 Cal (38% from Fat, 14% from Protein, 49% from Carb); 4 g Protein; 4 g Tot Fat; 1 g Sat Fat; 1 g Mono Fat; 13 g Carb; 0 g Fiber; 3 g Sugar; 44 mg Calcium; 1 mg Iron; 31 mg Sodium; 51 mg Cholesterol

YIELD: 10 servings

Apple Filling for Crêpes

5 large apples

1/4 cup plus 1 tablespoon nuts

1/4 cup plus 1 tablespoon raisins

1/2 cup plus 2 tablespoons apple butter

1/4 cup lemon juice

Cinnamon to taste

10 crêpes

Peel and slice the apples. Place them immediately in lemon juice to prevent browning. Poach the apples in the lemon juice plus enough water to cover them halfway (heightwise) and a little cinnamon. The apples should be barely tender. Remove from heat, strain, and set aside.

Spread 1 tablespoon apple butter on a warm crêpe. Add 2 ounces apples in the center. Sprinkle 1 1/2 teaspoon nuts, 1 1/2 teaspoon raisins, and cinnamon. Fold each side over the center and continue to cook for a minute. Serve immediately.

SERVING SIZE: 1 filled crêpe

PER SERVING: 87 Cal (22% from Fat, 7% from Protein, 71% from Carb); 2 g Protein; 2 g Tot Fat; 0 g Sat Fat; 1 g Mono Fat; 17 g Carb; 2 g Fiber; 12 g Sugar; 12 mg Calcium; 0 mg Iron; 3 mg Sodium; 0 mg Cholesterol (filling)

PER SERVING: 114 Cal (38% from Fat, 14% from Protein, 49% from Carb); 4 g Protein; 4 g Tot Fat; 1 g Sat Fat; 1 g Mono Fat; 13 g Carb; 0 g Fiber; 3 g Sugar; 44 mg Calcium; 1 mg Iron; 31 mg Sodium; 51 mg Cholesterol (crêpe)

YIELD: 10 servings

Strawberry Filling for Crêpes

Spread 1 tablespoon preserves on a warm crêpe. Add 2 ounces strawberries in the center. Fold each side over the center and continue to cook for a minute. Serve immediately.

1 1/3 pounds strawberries, trimmed and thinly sliced

10 tablespoons blackcurrant or boysenberry preserves

10 crêpes

SERVING SIZE: 1 filled crêpe

PER SERVING: 78 Cal (2% from Fat, 3% from Protein, 95% from Carb); 1 g Protein; 0 g Tot Fat; 0 g Sat Fat; 0 g Mono Fat; 19 g Carb; 1 g Fiber; 13 g Sugar; 14 mg Calcium; 0 mg Iron; 7 mg Sodium; 0 mg Cholesterol (filling)

PER SERVING: 114 Cal (38% from Fat, 14% from Protein, 49% from Carb); 4 g Protein; 4 g Tot Fat; 1 g Sat Fat; 1 g Mono Fat; 13 g Carb; 0 g Fiber; 3 g Sugar; 44 mg Calcium; 1 mg Iron; 31 mg Sodium; 51 mg Cholesterol (crêpe)

YIELD: 10 servings

Chocolate and Nut Filling for Crêpes

Mix the cocoa powder with the evaporated milk. Blend in the honey and almond butter until smooth. If needed, microwave for 5 seconds to help mix smoothly.

Spread 1 1/2 tablespoons chocolate filling on a warm crêpe. Fold each side over the center and continue to cook for 1 minute. Serve immediately.

2 tablespoons cocoa powder
6 tablespoons evaporated low-fat milk
4 teaspoons honey
3 1/2 ounces almond butter
10 crêpes

You may substitute low-fat milk for the evaporated low-fat milk.

This spread can also be used for bread, crackers, celery, muffin, filling, etc.

SERVING SIZE: 1 filled crêpe

PER SERVING: 81 Cal (61% from Fat, 11% from Protein, 28% from Carb); 2 g Protein; 6 g Tot Fat; 1 g Sat Fat; 4 g Mono Fat; 6 g Carb; 1 g Fiber; 3 g Sugar; 56 mg Calcium; 1 mg Iron; 12 mg Sodium; 0 mg Cholesterol (filling)

PER SERVING: 114 Cal (38% from Fat, 14% from Protein, 49% from Carb); 4 g Protein; 4 g Tot Fat; 1 g Sat Fat; 1 g Mono Fat; 13 g Carb; 0 g Fiber; 3 g Sugar; 44 mg Calcium; 1 mg Iron; 31 mg Sodium; 51 mg Cholesterol (crêpe)

YIELD: 10 servings

Poires au Muscat Noir
(POACHED PEARS WITH BLACK MUSCAT)

2 large ripe pears (Bosc)
1 1/2 tablespoons honey
12 ounces black Muscat wine
1/2 orange
1/2 lemon
1 cinnamon stick
1 teaspoon vanilla extract
1 teaspoon ground cardamom

Remove a large piece of the lemon peel and set aside. Juice the lemon and set aside. Remove a large piece of the orange peel and set aside. Juice the orange and set aside.

Peel, halve, and core the pears. Place them in a bowl and add the lemon juice. Mix well to prevent browning.

In a saucepan combine the wine, peels, juices, cinnamon, vanilla, and cardamom. Bring to a simmer over medium heat. Add the pears and simmer until tender when pierced with a knife, about 25 to 30 minutes. Remove the pears and set aside in a serving bowl. Reduce the wine to thicken (like syrup) and concentrate the flavors. Cool slightly, pass through a sieve, and add the sauce to the pears. Refrigerate and serve cold.

The dish may be refrigerated up to 2 days.

SERVING SIZE: 1/2 pear

PER SERVING: 210 Cal (1% from Fat, 3% from Protein, 96% from Carb); 1 g Protein; 0 g Tot Fat; 0 g Sat Fat; 0 g Mono Fat; 32 g Carb; 3 g Fiber; 19 g Sugar; 37 mg Calcium; 0 mg Iron; 10 mg Sodium; 0 mg Cholesterol

YIELD: 4 servings

Pommes au Four et Noix Grillées
(Baked Apples with Toasted Walnuts)

Preheat the broiler. Cover the bottom of a baking sheet with parchment paper. Add the walnuts and broil until slightly browned. Remove the walnuts from the sheet, cool, and chopped.

Preheat the oven to 400 degrees F.

4 apples

3 tablespoons orange preserves

4 tablespoons Chardonnay wine
(apple and citrus flavors)

4 teaspoons walnuts

Wash and core the apples, being careful not to break through the bottom of the apples. Place them in a baking pan that is just the right size to keep the apples close to each other. Put 1 teaspoon of preserves in the cavity of each apple. Pour 1 tablespoon of wine into the cavity of each apple. Add a little hot water in the pan (1/4 inch). Cover the pan with aluminum foil and bake for 20 minutes. Remove cover and baste with the liquid in the pan. Continue baking uncovered for 4 to 5 minutes. If necessary, add a little more water.

Place each apple in a serving dish. Scrape particles from the pan and transfer the liquid to a saucepan. Blend the liquid with the remaining preserves and bring to boil over high heat. Pour over the apples, sprinkle with the walnuts, and serve immediately.

Serving Size: 1 apple

Per Serving: 156 Cal (11% from Fat, 2% from Protein, 87% from Carb); 1 g Protein; 2 g Tot Fat; 0 g Sat Fat; 0 g Mono Fat; 34 g Carb; 4 g Fiber; 25 g Sugar; 17 mg Calcium; 0 mg Iron; 7 mg Sodium; 0 mg Cholesterol

Yield: 4 servings

Salade d'Oranges au Champagne
(ORANGE SALAD WITH CHAMPAGNE)

8 large oranges

3 tablespoons orange
blossom honey

1 1/2 cups water

1 teaspoon coriander
seeds (optional)

1 cup dry Champagne

2 tablespoons Grand Marnier

Peel and slice the oranges. Do not leave any white membranes on the oranges, as they have a bitter taste.

Cook the honey, coriander seeds (optional), and water in a saucepan over high heat for approximately 10 minutes to end up with 1 cup. Strain, place in a large bowl, and set aside to cool. Mix in the Champagne and Grand Marnier. Add the orange slices and refrigerate at least an hour.

SERVING SIZE: 1 orange

PER SERVING: 142 Cal (2% from Fat, 5% from Protein, 93% from Carb); 2 g Protein; 0 g Tot Fat; 0 g Sat Fat; 0 g Mono Fat; 30 g Carb; 4 g Fiber; 25 g Sugar; 73 mg Calcium; 0 mg Iron; 3 mg Sodium; 0 mg Cholesterol

YIELD: 8 servings

Marie's Oatmeal Cookies

Preheat the oven to 350 degrees F. Prepare a couple of cookie sheets covered with a Silpat or parchment paper.

Mix the almond meal, brown sugar, baking powder, baking soda, and salt. Blend in the egg and the preserves. Melt the butter and let cool for a minute.

Add the quick oats to the almond mixture and mix well. Finish by incorporating the melted butter.

Scoop out 1 tablespoon of dough onto the cookie sheet. Repeat, placing 3 inches apart to allow for spreading. Refrigerate for 20 minutes. Bake for 12 minutes or until golden brown. Let cool before transferring to a cooling rack.

7 ounces almond meal
1 cup quick oats
3/4 cup brown sugar
1 egg
1/4 teaspoon salt
2 ounces butter
2 ounces apricot preserves
1 1/2 teaspoons baking powder
3/4 teaspoon baking soda

This type of cookie will be moist. Don't store for more than 2 days at room temperature. They absorb moisture quickly and become very soggy. The best way to store them is to freeze immediately after they cool down. Defrost at room temperature when needed, for about half an hour.

You may add 1/2 cup of raisins, dry fruits, coconut, chocolate chips, chopped dates, nuts, or a combination of various ingredients. Remember any of these ingredients will add calories to the original recipe.

You may also add 1 teaspoon cinnamon and/or 1/2 teaspoon allspice.

You may substitute the brown sugar with 1/2 cup honey. Increase baking soda to 1 teaspoon and add 3/4 cup almond meal to balance moisture and texture. However, be aware that the cookie will not keep as well.

SERVING SIZE: 1 cookie

PER SERVING: 123 Cal (46% from Fat, 9% from Protein, 44% from Carb); 3 g Protein; 7 g Tot Fat; 2 g Sat Fat; 3 g Mono Fat; 14 g Carb; 2 g Fiber; 9 g Sugar; 48 mg Calcium; 1 mg Iron; 101 mg Sodium; 5 mg Cholesterol

YIELD: 24 servings

7

Specialties from the Chefs of Saint-Tropez

Aïgo Boulido
(GARLIC AND SAGE SOUP)

Chef Gui Alinat - Provence - Tampa, Florida

In a deep saucepan combine the water, garlic, and sage. Bring to a boil over high heat. Reduce heat and simmer 20 minutes.

Using a slotted spoon, remove the bunch of sage leaves. With an electric hand blender, blend the water and garlic together, right in the stock pot. Sprinkle with salt and pepper to taste. Remove from heat. Infuse the Italian parsley, bay leaf, and thyme for 15 minutes. Remove the bay leaf and thyme.

Prepare 6 soup bowls and place 2 croutons in the bottom of each bowl. Bring the soup back to a simmer. One at a time, break the eggs into a small bowl, and slip into the soup. Cook for 2 minutes. The yolks must remain soft. Transfer each egg from the soup on top of the 2 croutons. Pour some soup over the egg and croutons. Drizzle with 1 tablespoon olive oil and serve immediately.

8 cups of water
30 garlic cloves, peeled
10 fresh sage leaves, tied in a bunch
6 eggs
12 round croutons, made from toasted sourdough baguette
2 tablespoons of fresh Italian parsley, chopped
1 bay leaf
1 sprig of fresh thyme
6 tablespoons of a fruity extra virgin olive oil
Salt and pepper to taste

This recipe is very simple and relies on the quality of its ingredients. Choose your best estate olive oil, organic eggs, sea salt or "fleur de sel," freshly ground pepper, and fresh herbs.

"Aïgo Boulido" is known in Provence as a healthy, medicinal soup. The high concentration of vitamin C present in garlic and the natural benefits of sage make it a favorite for birthing mothers, stomach aches, and hangovers.

SERVING SIZE: 1/6 recipe

PER SERVING: 330 Cal (56% from Fat, 14% from Protein, 30% from Carb); 12 g Protein; 21 g Tot Fat; 4 g Sat Fat; 12 g Mono Fat; 25 g Carb; 1 g Fiber; 2 g Sugar; 124 mg Calcium; 3 mg Iron; 261 mg Sodium; 246 mg Cholesterol

YIELD: 6 servings

Tuna Carpaccio with Pistachios

Chef Gui Alinat - Provence - Tampa, Florida

Place a 10-inch by 10-inch piece of plastic wrap on a cutting board. Drizzle 1 teaspoon of olive oil onto the plastic wrap. Place one piece of tuna on top of wrap and drizzle 1 teaspoon of olive oil on top of tuna. Place an identical piece of plastic wrap on top of the tuna. With a kitchen mallet, gently pound tuna to paper thin, ensuring the consistency of the tuna is the same thinness. Repeat with remaining tuna, refrigerate, and set aside.

Gently peel plastic off of the tuna slices and place on serving platter. Drizzle 1 teaspoon olive oil on top of tuna, lemon juice, basil, salt, pepper, pistachios, and serve immediately.

Four 1-ounce pieces of sashimi-grade tuna
2 tablespoons pistachios, chopped
3 tablespoons fresh basil, chopped
3 tablespoons extra virgin olive oil
2 teaspoons lemon juice
Salt and pepper to taste

SERVING SIZE: 1/4 recipe

PER SERVING: 153 Cal (77% from Fat, 19% from Protein, 4% from Carb); 7 g Protein; 13 g Tot Fat; 2 g Sat Fat; 9 g Mono Fat; 1 g Carb; 0 g Fiber; 0 g Sugar; 10 mg Calcium; 1 mg Iron; 12 mg Sodium; 11 mg Cholesterol

YIELD: 4 servings

Caviar d'Aubergine
(Eggplant Caviar)

Chef Stéphane Furlan - Restaurant La Litote -
Vence, France

Preheat the oven to 350 degrees F.

Mince the thyme and keep the bare branches. Wash and slice the eggplants lengthwise. Score the slices with diagonal cuts from one end to the other and repeat from the other side. Place the slices on a baking pan. Spread the garlic slices, minced thyme, and thyme branches. Sprinkle with the olive oil and season to taste. Bake for 40 to 45 minutes or until tender. Discard the thyme branches. In a food processor purée the eggplant flesh, garlic, capers, herbs, and adjust seasonings.

5 1/2 pounds eggplants

5 garlic cloves, peeled and thinly sliced

1 cup olive oil

4 thyme branches

1 3/4 ounces capers

2 ounces anchovy fillets in oil

1 bunch fresh cilantro

1 bunch fresh basil

1 french baguette

Salt and pepper to taste

Preheat the oven to 450 degrees F. Slice the baguette diagonally. Place the slices on a baking sheet and bake until golden brown, which should take just a minute or two. Top each slice with some eggplant caviar, sprinkle with freshly grind pepper, and add half a piece of anchovy right in the center.

SERVING SIZE: 1 slice

PER SERVING: 277 Cal (70% from Fat, 7% from Protein, 23% from Carb); 5 g Protein; 23 g Tot Fat; 3 g Sat Fat; 16 g Mono Fat; 17 g Carb; 9 g Fiber; 6 g Sugar; 52 mg Calcium; 1 mg Iron; 383 mg Sodium; 5 mg Cholesterol

YIELD: 10 servings

Tomates en Millefeuilles
(TOMATOES NAPOLEON)

Chef Stéphane Furlan - Restaurant La Litote - Vence, France

For the marinade: In a bowl mix the garlic, oil, balsamic vinegar, herbs, shallots, and season to taste. Set aside for later use.

For the pesto: In a blender mix the capers, herbs, garlic, shallot, oil, and season to taste. Set aside for later use.

For the Napoleon: Make a small X incision on the top and bottom of the tomatoes. Blanch the tomatoes for 20 seconds. Place in ice-cold water to stop the cooking process. Peel the tomatoes. Slice the tomatoes and mozzarella, approximately 1/4 inch. Dip 4 slices of tomatoes in the marinade and brush 4 slices mozzarella with the pesto. Build the napoleon by alternating starting with a tomato slice and finishing with the mozzarella. Repeat to build 10 Napoleons. Refrigerate for 10 to 15 minutes or until cold. Serve each Napoleon on a bed of mesclun greens and sprinkle with 1 tablespoon pesto.

FOR THE NAPOLEON:
5 1/2 pounds tomatoes
2 pounds fresh buffalo mozzarella (skim milk)
6 ounces mesclun greens

FOR THE MARINADE:
3 garlic cloves, minced
1 cup olive oil
1 3/4 ounces balsamic vinegar
1 bunch fresh cilantro, chopped
1 bunch fresh basil, chopped
1 bunch fresh chervil, chopped
3/4 ounce shallots, minced

FOR THE PESTO:
1 3/4 ounces capers
1 bunch fresh basil
1 bunch fresh chervil
5 garlic cloves
1 ounce shallots
2 cups olive oil
Salt and pepper to taste

SERVING SIZE: 1/10 recipe

PER SERVING: 867 Cal (81% from Fat, 11% from Protein, 8% from Carb); 25 g Protein; 80 g Tot Fat; 18 g Sat Fat; 52 g Mono Fat; 17 g Carb; 3 g Fiber; 2 g Sugar; 738 mg Calcium; 2 mg Iron; 735 mg Sodium; 58 mg Cholesterol

YIELD: 10 servings

Gratin d'Aubergines
(Eggplant au Gratin)

Chef Jean-André Charial - Oustau de Baumanière - Les Baux de Provence, France

4 eggplants
6 ounces olive oil
1 bunch fresh basil
Bread crumbs
4 1/4 pounds tomatoes
1 onion, minced
3 garlic cloves, peeled
4 tablespoons olive oil
1 tablespoon sugar
1 tablespoon tomato paste
1 bunch basil
3 sprigs parsley
1 thyme branch
1 bay leaf
Salt and pepper to taste

The ingredients can be prepared a few hours before baking the gratin.

Prepare a baking dish with 3 cm of water (bain-marie). Place in the oven and heat the oven to the highest possible temperature. To avoid boiling during the cooking process, just place a piece of newspaper folded in half on the bottom of the baking dish.

Make a small X incision on the top and bottom of the tomatoes. Blanch the tomatoes for 20 seconds. Place in ice-cold water to stop the cooking process. Peel, seed, and dice the tomatoes.

Heat the oil in a saucepan over medium heat. Add the garlic cloves and sauté until golden brown. Add the onion and sauté until translucent. Add the tomatoes, sugar, tomato paste, parsley, thyme, bay leaf, and season to taste. Cook for an hour on low heat. Towards the end of cooking, add the basil.

To prepare the gratin: Peel the eggplants and slice lengthwise (approximately 1/8 inch). Heat the oil in a fryer pan and fry the eggplant slices on both sides until golden brown. Proceed by batches drying the slices immediately on paper towels.

Brush oil on the bottom of a gratin dish. Spread 1/4 inch of tomato mixture. Cover with eggplant slices and sprinkle with basil. Spread another layer of tomato and eggplant slices. Spread the remaining tomato mixture and cover with bread crumbs. Bake au bain-marie for 15 minutes and serve immediately.

SERVING SIZE: 1/8 recipe

PER SERVING: 371 Cal (66% from Fat, 5% from Protein, 29% from Carb); 5 g Protein; 29 g Tot Fat; 4 g Sat Fat; 21 g Mono Fat; 28 g Carb; 11 g Fiber; 8 g Sugar; 40 mg Calcium; 2 mg Iron; 45 mg Sodium; 0 mg Cholesterol

YIELD: 8 servings

Poached Red Mullet with Basil Sauce

Chef Jean-André Charial - Oustau de Baumanière - Les Baux de Provence, France

For the sauce: The sauce should be made the night before, since it is essential to blend the flavors. It can be made up to 2 or 3 days in advance.

Make a small X incision on the top and bottom of the tomatoes. Blanch the tomatoes for 20 seconds. Place in ice-cold water to stop the cooking process. Peel, seed, and finely chop the tomatoes. Place the tomatoes and herbs in a bowl and barely cover with olive oil. Add the garlic, vinegar, and season to taste. Refrigerate until use.

For the nage: Place all the ingredients in a large saucepan or fish kettle, add 3 quarts water, and season to taste. Bring to a boil and simmer for 30 minutes.

For the fish: While the nage is cooking, scale the fish but do not gut (the liver is a delicacy). Place a slice of orange, a slice of lemon, and a bay leaf on each fish. Wrap the fish individually in foil.

Once the nage is ready, place the fish foils in the nage and cook for 10 minutes. The fish should still be firm and hold its shape. Unwrap the fish and arrange on a serving dish with the orange and lemon slices. Serve the sauce on the side.

A nage is an aromatic broth in which seafood is cooked.

FOR THE FISH:
Four 6-ounce whole red mullets
4 orange slices
4 lemon slices
4 bay leaves

FOR THE NAGE:
9 ounces onions, chopped in rounds
14 ounces carrots, chopped in rounds
5 ounces celery, sliced in matchsticks
1 leek, green part only, chopped
1 garlic head, peeled and crushed
1/2 cup white wine vinegar
2 cups dry white wine
1/2 lemon
1 sprig thyme
1 bay leaf

FOR THE SAUCE:
6 ounces ripe plum tomatoes
20 basil leaves, chopped
5 tarragon leaves, chopped
5 sprigs parsley, chopped
Extra virgin olive oil
1 garlic clove, minced
3 drops sherry vinegar
Salt and pepper to taste

SERVING SIZE: One 6-ounce red mullet

PER SERVING: 502 Cal (15% from Fat, 33% from Protein, 52% from Carb); 39 g Protein; 8 g Tot Fat; 2 g Sat Fat; 2 g Mono Fat; 62 g Carb; 18 g Fiber; 11 g Sugar; 348 mg Calcium; 5 mg Iron; 229 mg Sodium; 83 mg Cholesterol

YIELD: 4 servings

La Daurade aux Amandes et Senteurs de Fleurs du Jardin
(SEA BREAM WITH ALMONDS AND EDIBLE FLOWERS)

Chef Jacques Chibois - La Bastide Saint-Antoine - Grasse, France

Four 5-ounce sea bream fillets
6 tablespoons olive oil
1 onion, sliced
1 garlic clove, minced
2 fresh dill branches
1 lemon
1 teaspoon fennel seeds
6 ounces fresh green beans, trimmed
1 yellow squash, cut into strips
1 bunch fresh cilantro, minced
1 ounce sliced almonds
1 bunch of edible flowers such as rose petal, nasturtium, wisteria, acacia, violet, and broom
Salt and pepper to taste

For the sauce: Grate 1 teaspoon of lemon zest and set aside for later use.

Heat 2 tablespoons of oil in a saucepan over high heat. Add the onion and sauté until translucent. Add 1 cup water, the garlic, dill branches, and season to taste. Reduce heat and simmer for 15 minutes. Remove the dill branches and transfer to a mixer. Add 2 tablespoons oil, lemon zest, a little of lemon juice, and purée. Transfer to a saucepan and add the fennel seeds. Bring to simmer over medium heat and continue to cook 1 minute. Remove from heat and set aside.

For the vegetables: Heat a pan with just enough water to cover the beans, 1 teaspoon salt, and bring to boil over high heat. Add the green beans and cook until tender.

Meanwhile heat another pan with water and bring to boil over high heat. Blanch the squash quickly and strain immediately.

For the fish: Heat 2 tablespoons oil in a large sauté pan over high heat. Add the sea bream fillets and sauté until golden brown. Carefully turn over, season to taste, and sprinkle with lemon juice. Reduce heat and cook until the flesh starts to flake.

Bring the prepared sauce to boil, add the cilantro, and adjust seasonings.

Place the green beans and squash on a platter. Top with the fish fillets. Sprinkle with almonds, a little bit of the sauce, and the edible flowers. Pour the remaining sauce in a sauceboat and serve immediately.

SERVING SIZE: One 5-ounce sea bream fillet

PER SERVING: 396 Cal (56% from Fat, 31% from Protein, 13% from Carb); 31 g Protein; 26 g Tot Fat; 3 g Sat Fat; 18 g Mono Fat; 13 g Carb; 5 g Fiber; 4 g Sugar; 113 mg Calcium; 3 mg Iron; 82 mg Sodium; 52 mg Cholesterol

YIELD: 4 servings

Fraicheur de Brugnon aux Framboises à la Verveine Fraiche
(Nectarine with Raspberries and Fresh Verbena)

Chef Jacques Chibois - La Bastide Saint-Antoine - Grasse, France

For the nectarines: Peel and cut the nectarines into segments. Bring to a boil 2 cups water, 3 1/2 ounces sugar, 2 lemon peels, and 1 vanilla bean (split in half, scrape the center, and add all to the water) in a saucepan over high heat. Reduce a little bit to concentrate the flavors. Add the nectarine segments and simmer for 2 minutes. Strain with a bowl underneath to retain the liquid. Set aside 1 cup of the cooking liquid and add the minced verbena leaves to flavor the sauce.

For the coulis: Place the raspberries, sugar, and juice of 1/2 lemon in a blender. Liquefy and strain. Bring to a simmer over medium heat. Remove from heat and set aside to cool. Transfer to a sauceboat, cool down, and refrigerate.

For the Chantilly: With a hand mixer, beat the heavy cream adding the sugar halfway through. Mix in the verbena leaves.

To assemble: You will need 4 plates. Place some nectarines in a circle on the center of the plate. Spoon some Chantilly on the middle of the nectarines. Form a ring with the raspberries around the Chantilly. Drizzle some sauce and raspberry coulis. Top with a verbena leaf.

FOR THE NECTARINES:

4 nectarines

2 cups water

3 1/2 ounces sugar

2 lemon peels

1 vanilla bean

10 verbena leaves, minced

FOR THE COULIS:

4 ounces raspberries

1 ounce sugar

juice of 1/2 lemon

FOR THE CHANTILLY:

1 cup heavy cream

1 3/4 tablespoons sugar

10 verbena leaves, minced

14 ounces fresh raspberries

FOR THE DÉCOR:

4 verbena leaves

SERVING SIZE: 1 nectarine

PER SERVING: 377 Cal (28% from Fat, 4% from Protein, 69% from Carb); 4 g
Protein; 12 g Tot Fat; 7 g Sat Fat; 3 g Mono Fat; 69 g Carb; 11 g Fiber; 54 g
Sugar; 70 mg Calcium; 1 mg Iron; 15 mg Sodium; 41 mg Cholesterol

YIELD: 4 servings

Fillets de Sole Poelés au Velouté de Coco Blanc
(SOLE FILLETS WITH WHITE BEANS VELOUTÉ)

Chef Xavier Mathieu - Hostellerie Le Phébus - Gordes, France

FOR THE FISH:
Six 5-ounce fillets of sole
5 ounces pot-au-feu broth or beef broth

FOR THE SAUCE:
5 ounces white beans
1 bunch fresh thyme branches
1 garlic clove, crushed
1 onion, diced small
1 carrot, diced small
1 lime
1/2 lemon

FOR THE ARTICHOKES:
6 artichokes
1 ounce olive oil
5 ounces pot-au-feu broth or beef broth
1 bunch fresh cilantro, minced
3 juniper berries, crushed
18 black olives
Salt and pepper to taste

For the sauce: Soak the beans in water overnight.

Place the beans in a pan and cover with water. Add the garlic, onion, carrot, and 1 thyme branch. Bring to boil over high heat. Reduce heat and simmer until tender (40 to 45 minutes). Remove the thyme and purée the beans. Return to the pan; add 5 ounces broth, and the thyme branches. Bring to a boil over medium heat. Remove from heat, cover, and infuse for 20 minutes. Pass through a sieve. Place in a blender; add the lime and lemon juices. Blend until smooth and season to taste.

For the artichokes: Snap off the stem of the artichokes. Cut off and discard the leaves until you reach the inner core. Cut off the top leaving about 1 inch. Trim the bottom and remove the tough green parts. You should end up with a smooth round bottom. Cut each bottom into 8 pieces. Heat the oil in a saucepan over medium heat. Add the artichoke pieces and sauté for a couple of minutes, but do not brown. Add the broth, juniper berries, and bring to a boil. Boil at high temperature for 10 minutes. Strain reserving the cooking liquid. Add the cilantro, black olives, and season to taste. If necessary moisten with the cooking liquid.

For the fish: Preheat a steamer. Add the fillets and cook until the flesh barely starts to flake. Place the fillets in a serving platter and pour over some sauce. Spread the vegetables nicely on top, finish by adding a few pinches of cilantro, and serve immediately.

SERVING SIZE: One 5-ounce fillet of sole

PER SERVING: 401 Cal (19% from Fat, 45% from Protein, 35% from Carb); 47 g Protein; 9 g Tot Fat; 1 g Sat Fat; 5 g Mono Fat; 37 g Carb; 13 g Fiber; 3 g Sugar; 176 mg Calcium; 5 mg Iron; 655 mg Sodium; 96 mg Cholesterol

YIELD: 6 servings

Effeuille de Poissons en Salade
(Fish Petals Salad)

Chef Yves Rouet - Restaurant Le Girelier - Saint-Tropez, France

For the shallots compote: Make a small X incision on the top and bottom of the tomato. Blanch the tomato for 20 seconds. Remove and place in ice cold water to stop the cooking process. Peel, seed, and mince the tomatoes. Mince the shallots, garlic, and parsley. Heat 1 tablespoon olive oil in a large skillet over medium heat. Add the shallots, garlic, tomato, vinegar, parsley, and bring to a boil. Reduce heat and simmer for 30 minutes. Remove from heat and set aside.

For the salad: In a bowl mix mesclun greens, lemon juice, and 2 tablespoons olive oil. Add salt and pepper to taste. Set aside.

Thinly slice the fish into rose petals and sprinkle with salt and pepper. Heat 1 tablespoon olive oil in a large skillet over medium heat. Add the fish petals and sauté quickly. Turn over the petals and continue to sauté until cooked through.

To assemble: Divide the mesclun greens over four plates, piling high in the center. Arrange the fish petals around the outside of the plate. Spoon out a little warm shallots compote over each petal. Top with 1 chervil branch and 3 mussels per plate (optional).

For best result, use sushi grade fish.

FOR THE SALAD:
4 ounces mesclun greens
1 tablespoon lemon juice
3 tablespoons olive oil
3 1/2 ounces salmon
3 1/2 ounces monkfish
3 1/2 ounces swordfish
3 1/2 ounces Ahi tuna
12 cooked mussels with
    shell (about 4 ounces)
    (optional)
4 fresh chervil branches
Salt and pepper to taste

**FOR THE SHALLOTS
    COMPOTE:**
1 large tomato
4 large shallots, skin re-
    moved
1 1/2 garlic cloves
1 large fresh parsley branch
1 tablespoon olive oil
1 tablespoon red wine vine-
    gar
Salt and pepper to taste

PER SERVING: 340 Cal (11% from Fat, 28% from Protein, 61% from Carb); 27 g Protein; 5 g Tot Fat; 1 g Sat Fat; 3 g Mono Fat; 59 g Carb; 0 g Fiber; 54 g Sugar; 57 mg Calcium; 1 mg Iron; 146 mg Sodium; 61 mg Cholesterol

YIELD: 4 Servings

Tarte Fine de Primeurs Tendres
(THIN TART WITH PRIME TENDER VEGETABLES)

Chef Arnaud Donckele - Résidence de la Pinède - Saint-Tropez, France

For the tart base: Roll out thinly the dough and place on a greased baking sheet. Top with parchment paper and another greased baking sheet, so the dough does not rise during the cooking process. Cook in the oven according to the type of dough.

For the filling: Preheat the oven to 175 degrees F. Make a small X incision on the top and bottom of the tomatoes. Blanch the tomatoes for 20 seconds. Remove and place in ice-cold water to stop the cooking process. Peel, halve, and seed. Place a parchment paper over a baking sheet and spread the tomato halves on the baking sheet (cut side up). Slice some garlic cloves to end up with 20 slices. On each tomato half, place 1 garlic slice, 1 rosemary branch, and sprinkle a little olive oil. Place in the oven and bake for 1 hour 30 minutes. Remove garlic, rosemary, dice, and set aside.

FOR THE TART BASE:
8 ounces of your favorite dough (tart, pizza, puff pastry, or any thin bread recipe)

FOR THE TART TOPPINGS:
10 Roma tomatoes
12 small purple artichokes, trimmed
2 baby zucchinis, trimmed
12 purple asparagus, trimmed
32 green beans, trimmed
1 1/2 ounces green peas
1 1/2 ounces cooked white beans
A few celery branches (with bright yellow leaves)
4 red radishes
1 garlic head
1 heart of Romaine (about 4 ounces)
4 chicory leaves
1 small bunch of edible flowers
    such as nasturtium
40 mesclun leaves (about 1 ounce)
12 garlic chives
22 small rosemary branches
16 small savory leaves
3 1/2 ounces fresh tuna filet
2 hard boiled eggs, sliced
2/3 ounces piquillos peppers
2/3 ounces pitted black olives
3 1/2 ounces reduced balsamic vinegar
1/4 cup veal or vegetable stock
Olive oil
Salt and pepper to taste

Heat a little olive oil in a sauté pan over medium heat. Add the artichokes, 2 garlic cloves, and 2 rosemary branches. Remove the artichokes; add the zucchini, asparagus, celery, beans, peas, and enough stock to moisten. Cook until tender and season to taste.

Meanwhile, broil or grill the tuna fillet to desired doneness. Thinly slice the radishes, artichokes, olives, and piquillos peppers. Trim the celery branches, so they end up looking like small fans.

For the anchovy tempura: Preheat a fryer. Mix the tempura with the water, chlorophyll, and minced rosemary. Dip the anchovy fillets in the tempura mixture and immediately fry them until golden brown. Remove and set aside on a paper towel to absorb excess grease.

For the tuna vinaigrette: In a blender mix the tuna, egg yolk, vinegar, and season to taste.

To assemble: Place the cooked dough on a platter. Spread the roasted tomatoes, top with the remaining vegetables and filling ingredients harmoniously. Make sure the salad leaves and celery leaves are pointing up to give height. Pour over the vinaigrette, sprinkle with nasturtiums, and serve with the tempura anchovies on the side.

ANCHOVY TEMPURA

12 fresh small anchovies, head removed
and filleted
2 1/2 ounces tempura
2 1/2 ounces water
1/3 ounce chlorophyll
1 rosemary branch

TUNA VINAIGRETTE

2 1/2 ounces Ventresca tuna, premium belly fillets in olive oil, or bonito tuna
1 egg yolk
7 ounces olive oil
2 ounces aged wine vinegar (if not available, substitute regular wine vinegar
Salt and pepper

SERVING SIZE: 1/4 recipe

PER SERVING: 890 Cal (52% from Fat, 21% from Protein, 27% from Carb); 48 g Protein; 54 g Tot Fat; 9 g Sat Fat; 35 g Mono Fat; 63 g Carb; 21 g Fiber; 15 g Sugar; 536 mg Calcium; 14 mg Iron; 417 mg Sodium; 136 mg Cholesterol

YIELD: 4 servings

List of Recipes

CHAPTER 1 **Breakfasts**

CHAPTER 2 **Fish Entrees**

CHAPTER 3 Meat Entrees

CHAPTER 5 Snacks and Side Dishes

Conclusion

By now you should feel at home with the ideas covered in *The Saint-Tropez Diet*. You have learned that a diet rich in omega-3 fatty acids will give your body the message to burn fat, particularly when these fatty acids are paired with fruits and vegetables rich in vitamin A. You've read about the hidden power of certain superfoods to increase your energy level and protect you against disease and inflammation. You've also learned about the myths of dieting that can derail your efforts to lose weight. You may have even read through some of the delicious recipes that will help you lose weight.

As you prepare to journey to Saint-Tropez (at least in spirit), you'll want to review the four basic principles that will guide you toward your weight loss goals. First, you should remember to stock your refrigerator and pantry with foods loaded with healthy, unsaturated fats. These include fatty fish such as salmon, sardines, anchovies, and herring, which are high in omega-3 fatty acids. Walnuts and ground flaxseed are also high in omega-3s, along with walnut and flaxseed oil, so you should keep those on hand as well. In addition, you should have plenty of other healthy oils for cooking, such as olive oil and canola oil. Look to include one to two servings of these healthy oils into your diet every day.

Next, you'll need to eat more of the right kinds of fruits and vegetables, meaning those that are most colorful. Remember that boosting your omega-3 fatty acid intake is only half the battle. You'll need to pair those foods with lots of natural vitamin A found in yellow, orange, red, and green vegetables, such as pumpkin, tomatoes, carrots, squash, and broccoli.

Finally, you'll want to round out your shopping list with the kinds of foods that will help change your overall ratio of omega-3 to omega-6 fatty acids and with healthy nutraceuticals that will help keep your energy high while your body is shedding fat and toxins. Some diets might encourage you to turn to supplements to increase the level of antioxidants and omega-3 fatty acids. With the Saint-Tropez Diet, you won't need supplements because you'll be eating meals full of healthy foods such as apples, berries, nuts, whole grains, and dark green leafy vegetables. Each week, you'll be eating three or four servings of lean, grass-fed meats—and even a bit of whole milk to round out the nutritional spectrum.

Once you've done your shopping, you'll want to clean out the pantry. Get rid of all of those boxed and packaged foods that will sabotage the Saint-Tropez Diet. Most processed foods are loaded with chemicals, fillers, and emulsifiers with no nutritional value at all. Many of them are high in trans fat or just high in refined flours and omega-6 fatty acids that will prevent your body from burning fat as it should. Give up entirely on diet foods and "low-calorie" processed foods. They'll do nothing for you. Resolve to stay away from vending machine foods and deli foods that will keep you from losing weight and achieving the energy level that you want.

There's no need to get discouraged if you struggle at first to stick to this new way of eating. Remember that every meal, every snack offers an opportunity to make the right choices to improve your diet and your health. Every time you go to the store or the farmer's market, every time you walk into your kitchen, and every time you sit down to a meal, you are choosing to live a better life. Good luck.

References

CHAPTER 2 Improving on the Healthiest Diet in the World

Agatston A. *The South Beach Diet*. Rodale (2003).

Belleville J. "The French paradox: possible involvement of ethanol in the protective effect against cardiovascular diseases." *Nutrition*. (2002 Feb) 18(2):173-7.

Frankel EN et al., "Inhibition of oxidation of human low-density lipoprotein by phenolic substances in red wine." *Lancet*. (1993 April 24) 341(8852):1104.

Guiliano M. *French Women Don't Get Fat*. Random House (2004).

Keys A et al., "The diet and 15-year death rate in the seven countries study." *Am J Epidemiol*. (1986 Dec) 124(6):903-15.

Montignac M. *Eat Yourself Slim*. Alex & Lucas Publishing (2004).

Muoio DM and Newgard CB. "Obesity-related derangements in metabolic regulation." *Annu Rev Biochem*. (2006) 75:367-401.

Perricone N. *The Perricone Weight-Loss Diet*. Random House (2005).

Renaud S, de Lorgeril M, Delaye J, Guidollet J, Jacquard F, Mamelle N, Martin JL, Monjaud I, Salen P, Touboul P. "Cretan Mediterranean diet for prevention of coronary heart disease." *Am J Clin Nutr*. 61 (1995):(suppl.):1360S-1367S.

Richard JL. "Coronary risk factors. The French paradox." *Arch Mal Coeur Vaiss*. (1987 Apr) 80 Spec No:17-21.

Simopoulos AP. "The Mediterranean diets: What is so special about the diet of Greece? The scientific evidence." *J Nutr*. (2001 Nov) 131(11 Suppl):3065S-73S.

Simopoulos AP. "The traditional diet of Greece and cancer." *Eur J Cancer Prev*. (2004 June) 13(3):219-30.

Simopoulos AP and Robinson J. *The Omega Diet*. HarperCollins (1999).

Sun AY et al., "The 'French Paradox' and beyond: neuroprotective effects of polyphenols." *Free Radic Biol Med*. (2002 Feb 15) 32(4):314-8.

Tricopoulou A, Costacou T, Bamia C, Trichopoulos D. "Adherence to a Mediterranean diet and survival in a Greek population." *N Engl J Med*. (2003) 348:2599-608.

Willett WC. "The Mediterranean diet: science and practice." *Public Health Nutr*. (2006 Feb) 9(1A):105-10.

CHAPTER 3 The Good and the Bad of Fat

Agren JJ et al., "Fish diet, fish oil and docosahexaenoic acid rich oil lower fasting and postprandial plasma lipid levels." *Eur J Clin Nutr*. (1996 Nov) 50(11):765-71.

Belury MA, Mahon A, Banni S. "The conjugated linoleic acid (CLA) isomer, t10c12-CLA, is inversely associated with changes in body weight and serum leptin in subjects with type 2 diabetes mellitus." *J Nutr.* (2003 Jan) 133(1):257S-260S.

Brodie AE, Manning VA, Ferguson KR, Jewell DE, Hu CY. "Conjugated linoleic acid inhibits differentiation of pre- and post- confluent 3T3-L1 preadipocytes but inhibits cell proliferation only in preconfluent cells." *J Nutr.* (1999 Mar) 129(3):602-6.

Brown MJ, et al., "Carotenoid bioavailability is higher from salads ingested with full-fat than with fat-reduced salad dressings as measured with electrochemical detection." *Am J Clin Nutr.* (2004 Aug) 80(2):396-403.

"Dietary Reference Intake: Vitamins." Institute of Medicine of the National Academies. http://www.iom.edu/Object.File/Master/7/296/webtablevitamins.pdf (accessed 2006 Sept)

Dobrzyn P, Dobrzyn A, Miyazaki M, Cohen P, Asilmaz E, Hardie DG, Friedman JM, Ntambi JM. "Stearoyl-CoA desaturase 1 deficiency increases fatty acid oxidation by activating AMP-activated protein kinase in liver." *Proc Natl Acad Sci U S A.* (2004 Apr 27) 101(17):6409-14. Epub (2004 Apr 19).

Eaton SB. "The ancestral human diet: what was it and should it be a paradigm for contemporary nutrition?" *Proc Nutr Soc.* (2006 Feb) 65(1):1-6.

Faine LA et al., "Effects of olive oil and its minor constituents on serum lipids, oxidative stress, and energy metabolism in cardiac muscle." *Can J Physiol Pharmacol.* (2006 Feb) 84(2):239-45.

"Fats and Oils, Structures and Biology." www.lipidlibrary.co.uk (accessed 2006 Sept)

Fielding JM et al., "Increases in plasma lycopene concentration after consumption of tomatoes cooked with olive oil." *Asia Pac J Clin Nutr.* (2005) 14(2):131-6.

Fontani G et al., "Blood profiles, body fat and mood state in healthy subjects on different diets supplemented with Omega-3 polyunsaturated fatty acids." *Eur J Clin Invest.* (2005 Aug) 35(8):499-507

Fontani G et al., "Cognitive and physiological effects of Omega-3 polyunsaturated fatty acid supplementation in healthy subjects." *Eur J Clin Invest.* (2005 Nov) 35(11):691-9.

Gaullier JM et al., "Conjugated linoleic acid supplementation for 1 y reduces body fat mass in healthy overweight humans." *Am J Clin Nutr.* (2004 Jun) 79(6):1118-25.

Gaullier JM, Halse J, Hoye K, Kristiansen K, Fagertun H, Vik H, Gudmundsen O. "Supplementation with conjugated linoleic acid for 24 months is well tolerated by and reduces body fat mass in healthy, overweight humans." *J Nutr.* (2005 Apr) 135(4):778-84.

Harrison EH. "Mechanisms of digestion and absorption of dietary vitamin A." *Annu Rev Nutr.* (2005) 25:87-103.

Holguin F et al., "Cardiac autonomic changes associated with fish oil vs. soy oil supplementation in the elderly." *Chest.* (2005 Apr) 127(4):1102-7.

Kamphuis MM, Lejeune MP, Saris WH, Westerterp-Plantenga MS. "The effect of conjugated linoleic acid supplementation after weight loss on body weight regain, body composition, and resting metabolic rate in overweight subjects." *Int J Obes Relat Metab Disord*. (2003 Jul) 27(7):840-7.

Miyazaki M, Kim YC, Ntambi JM. "A lipogenic diet in mice with a disruption of the stearoyl-CoA desaturase 1 gene reveals a stringent requirement of endogenous monounsaturated fatty acids for triglyceride synthesis." *J Lipid Res*. (2001 Jul) 42(7):1018-24.

Moya-Camarena SY, Vanden Heuvel JP, Blanchard SG, Leesnitzer LA, Belury MA. "Conjugated linoleic acid is a potent naturally occurring ligand and activator of PPARalpha." *J Lipid Res*. (1999 Aug) 40(8):1426-33.

Moya-Camarena SY, Van den Heuvel JP, Belury MA. "Conjugated linoleic acid activates peroxisome proliferator-activated receptor alpha and beta subtypes but does not induce hepatic peroxisome proliferation in Sprague-Dawley rats." *Biochim Biophys Acta*. (1999 Jan 4) 1436(3):331-42.

Mulokozi G et al., "In vitro accessibility and intake of beta-carotene from cooked green leafy vegetables and their estimated contribution to vitamin A requirements." *Plant Foods Hum Nutr*. (2004 Winter) 59(1):1-9.

Ntambi JM, Miyazaki M, Dobrzyn A. "Regulation of stearoyl-CoA desaturase expression." *Lipids*. (2004 Nov):39(11):1061-5.

Perez-Jimenez F et al., "International conference on the healthy effect of virgin olive oil." *Eur J Clin Invest*. (2005 Jul) 35(7):421-4.

Ribaya-Mercado JD. "Influence of dietary fat on beta-carotene absorption and bioconversion into vitamin A." *Nutr Rev*. (2002 Apr) 60(4):104-10.

Riserus U, Vessby B, Arnlov J, Basu S. "Effects of cis-9,trans-11 conjugated linoleic acid supplementation on insulin sensitivity, lipid peroxidation, and proinflammatory markers in obese men." *Am J Clin Nutr*. (2004 Aug) 80(2):279-83.

Simopoulos AP and Salem N Jr. "N-3 fatty acids in eggs from range-fed Greek chickens." *N Engl J Med*. (1989 Nov 16) 321(20):1412.

Simopoulos AP. "The importance of the ratio of omega-6/omega-3 essential fatty acids." *Biomed Pharmacother*. (2002 Oct) 56(8):365-79.

Terpstra AH. "Effect of conjugated linoleic acid on body composition and plasma lipids in humans: an overview of the literature." *Am J Clin Nutr*. (2004 Mar) 79(3):352-61.

Tsuzuki T, Kawakami Y, Nakagawa K, Miyazawa T. "Conjugated docosahexaenoic acid inhibits lipid accumulation in rats." *J Nutr Biochem*. (2006 Aug) 17(8):518-24. Epub 10/25/05.

Tsuzuki T, Kawakami Y, Suzuki Y, Abe R, Nakagawa K, Miyazawa T. "Intake of conjugated eicosapentaenoic acid suppresses lipid accumulation in liver and epididymal adipose tissue in rats." *Lipids*. (2005 Nov) 40(11):1117-23.

Unlu NZ et al., "Carotenoid absorption from salad and salsa by humans is enhanced by the addition of avocado or avocado oil." *J Nutr*. (2005 Mar) 135(3):431-6.

Yang M, Cook ME. "Dietary conjugated linoleic acid decreased cachexia, macrophage tumor necrosis factor-alpha production, and modifies spleno-cyte cytokines production." *Exp Biol Med* (Maywood). (2003 Jan) 228(1):51-8.

Zhao G et al., "Dietary alpha-linolenic acid reduces inflammatory and lipid car-diovascular risk factors in hypercholesterolemic men and women." *J Nutr.* (2004 Nov) 134(11):2991-7.

Zhang L, Ge L, Tran T, Stenn K, Prouty SM. "Isolation and characterization of the human stearoyl-CoA desaturase gene promoter: requirement of a con-served CCAAT cis-element." *Biochem J.* (2001 Jul 1) 357(Pt 1):183-93.

CHAPTER 4 Turbocharging Your Fat-Burning Receptors

Bailey CJ. "Drugs on the horizon for diabesity." *Curr Diab Rep.* (2005 Oct) 5(5):353-9.

Clarke SD, Turini M, Jump DB, Abraham S, Reedy M. "Polyunsaturated fatty acid inhibition of fatty acid synthase transcription is independent of PPAR activation." *Z Ernahrungswiss.* (1998) 37 Suppl 1:14-20.

Clarke SD, Jump D. "Polyunsaturated fatty acids regulate lipogenic and peroxiso-mal gene expression by independent mechanisms." *Prostaglandins Leukot Es-sent Fatty Acids.* (1997 Jul):57(1):65-9. Review. Erratum in: *Prostaglandins Leukot Essent Fatty Acids* (1997 Oct) 57(4-5):526.

Delarue J, LeFoll C, Corporeau C, Lucas D. "N-3 long chain polyunsaturated fatty acids: a nutritional tool to prevent insulin resistance associated to type 2 diabetes and obesity?" *Reprod Nutr Dev.* (2004 May-Jun) 44(3):289-99.

Evans RM, Barish GD, Wang YX. "PPARs and the complex journey to obesity." *Nat Med.* (2004 Apr) 10(4):355-61.

Forman BM, Chen J, Evans RM. "Hypolipidemic drugs, polyunsaturated fatty acids, and eicosanoids are ligands for peroxisome proliferator-activated re-ceptors alpha and delta." *Proc Natl Acad Sci U S A.* (1997 Apr 29) 94(9):4312-7.

Jump DB, Clarke SD. "Regulation of gene expression by dietary fat." *Annu Rev Nutr.* (1999) 19:63-90.

Jump DB, Clarke SD, Thelen A, Liimatta M, Ren B, Badin MV. "Dietary fat, genes, and human health." *Adv Exp Med Biol.* (1997) 422:167-76. Review.

Lee CH, Olson P, Evans RM. "Minireview: lipid metabolism, metabolic diseases, and peroxisome proliferator-activated receptors." *Endocrinology.* (2003 Jun) 144(6):2201-7.

McCarthy TC, Pollak PT, Hanniman EA, Sinal CJ. "Disruption of hepatic lipid homeostasis in mice after amiodarone treatment is associated with peroxi-some proliferator-activated receptor-alpha target gene activation." *J Pharma-col Exp Ther.* (2004 Dec) 311(3):864-73. Epub (2004 Jul 20).

Mori TA, Burke V, Puddey IB, Shaw JE, Beilin LJ. "Effect of fish diets and weight loss on serum leptin concentration in overweight, treated-hypertensive sub-jects." *J Hypertens.* (2004 Oct) 22(10):1983-90.

Sampath H, Ntambi JM. "Polyunsaturated fatty acid regulation of gene expres-sion." *Nutr Rev.* (2004 Sep) 62(9):333-9.

Sesti G, Perego L, Cardellini M, Andreozzi F, Ricasoli C, Vedani P, Guzzi V, Marchi M, Paganelli M, Ferla G, Pontiroli AE, Hribal ML, Folli F. "Impact of common polymorphisms in candidate genes for insulin resistance and obesity on weight loss of morbidly obese subjects after laparoscopic adjustable gastric banding and hypocaloric diet." *J Clin Endocrinol Metab.* (2005 Sep) 90(9):5064-9. Epub 06/28/05. Erratum in: *J Clin Endocrinol Metab.* (2005 Oct) 90(10):5810.

Verreth W, De Keyzer D, Pelat M, Verhamme P, Ganame J, Bielicki JK, Mertens A, Quarck R, Benhabiles N, Marguerie G, Mackness B, Mackness M, Ninio E, Herregods MC, Balligand JL, Holvoet P. "Weight-loss-associated induction of peroxisome proliferator-activated receptor-alpha and peroxisome proliferator-activated receptor-gamma correlate with reduced atherosclerosis and improved cardiovascular function in obese insulin-resistant mice." *Circulation.* 2004 (Nov 16) 110(20):3259-69. Epub (2004 Nov 08).

Vidal-Puig AJ, Considine RV, Jimenez-Linan M, Werman A, Pories WJ, Caro JF, Flier JS. "Peroxisome proliferator-activated receptor gene expression in human tissues. Effects of obesity, weight loss, and regulation by insulin and glucocorticoids." *J Clin Invest.* (1997 May 15) 99(10):2416-22.

Vogels N, Mariman EC, Bouwman FG, Kester AD, Diepvens K, Westerterp-Plantenga MS. "Relation of weight maintenance and dietary restraint to peroxisome proliferator-activated receptor gamma2, glucocorticoid receptor, and ciliary neurotrophic factor polymorphisms." *Am J Clin Nutr.* (2005 Oct) 82(4):740-6.

CHAPTER 5 The Power of Nutraceuticals

Agarwal S, Hordvik S, Morar S. "Nutritional claims for functional foods and supplements." *Toxicology* (2006 Apr 3) 221(1):44-9. Epub (2006 Feb 8).

Barbaste M, Berke B, Dumas M, Soulet S, Delaunay JC, Castagnino C, Arnaud-inaud V, Cheze C, Vercauteren J. "Dietary antioxidants, peroxidation and cardiovascular risks." *J Nutr Health Aging* (2002 May) 6(3):209-23.

Bhuvaneswari V, Nagini S. "Lycopene: a review of its potential as an anticancer agent." *Curr Med Chem Anticancer Agents* (2005 Nov) 5(6):627-35.

Boyer J, Liu RH. "Apple phytochemicals and their health benefits." *Nutr J.* (2004 May 12):3:5.

Eberhardt MV, Lee CY, Liu RH. "Antioxidant activity of fresh apples." *Nature* (2000 Jun 22) 405(6789):903-4.

Engler MB, Engler MM. "The emerging role of flavonoid-rich cocoa and chocolate in cardiovascular health and disease." *Nutr Rev.* (2006 Mar) 64(3):109-18.

Fraser ML, Lee AH, Binns CW. "Lycopene and prostate cancer: emerging evidence." *Expert Rev Anticancer Ther.* (2005 Oct) 5(5):847-54.

Hamer M, Steptoe A. "Influence of specific nutrients on progression of ather osclerosis, vascular function, haemostasis and inflammation in coronary heart disease patients: a systematic review." *Br J Nutr.* (2006 May) 95(5):849-59.

Hardy G, Hardy I, Ball PA. "Nutraceuticals—a pharmaceutical viewpoint: part II." *Curr Opin Clin Nutr Metab Care* (2003 Nov) 6(6):661-71.

Higuera-Ciapara I, Felix-Valenzuela L, Goycoolea FM. "Astaxanthin: a review of its chemistry and applications." *Crit Rev Food Sci Nutr.* (2006) 46(2):185-96.

Iriti M, Faoro F. "Grape phytochemicals: A bouquet of old and new nutraceuticals for human health." *Med Hypotheses.* (2006) 67(4):833-8. Epub (2006 Jun 8).

Kovacs EM, Mela DJ. "Metabolically active functional food ingredients for weight control." *Obes Rev.* (2006 Feb) 7(1):59-78.

Krinsky NI, Landrum JT, Bone RA. "Biological mechanisms of the protective role of lutein and zeaxanthin in the eye." *Annu Rev Nutr.* (2003) 23:171-201. Epub (2003 Feb 27).

Liu RH, Liu J, Chen B. "Apples prevent mammary tumors in rats." *J Agric Food Chem.* (2005 Mar 23) 53(6):2341-3.

Liu RH. "Health benefits of fruit and vegetables are from additive and synergistic combinations of phytochemicals." *Am J Clin Nutr.* (2003 Sep) 78(3 Suppl):517S-520S.

Liu RH, Sun J. "Antiproliferative activity of apples is not due to phenolic-induced hydrogen peroxide formation." *J Agric Food Chem.* (2003 Mar 12) 51(6):1718-23.

Muhlhofer A, Mrosek S, Schlegel B, Trommer W, Rozario F, Bohles H, Schremmer D, Zoller WG, Biesalski HK. "High-dose intravenous vitamin C is not associated with an increase of pro-oxidative biomarkers." *Eur J Clin Nutr.* (2004 Aug) 58(8):1151-8.

Nichenametla SN, Taruscio TG, Barney DL, Exon JH. "A review of the effects and mechanisms of polyphenolics in cancer." *Crit Rev Food Sci Nutr.* 2006;46(2):161-83.

Podmore ID, Griffiths HR, Herbert KE, Mistry N, Mistry P, Lunec J. "Vitamin C exhibits pro-oxidant properties." *Nature* (1998) 392:559.

Rajesha J, Murthy KN, Kumar MK, Madhusudhan B, Ravishankar GA. "Antioxidant potentials of flaxseed by in vivo model." *J Agric Food Chem.* (2006 May 31) 54(11):3794-9.

Ribaya-Mercado JD, Blumberg JB. "Lutein and zeaxanthin and their potential roles in disease prevention." *J Am Coll Nutr.* (2004 Dec) 23(6 Suppl):567S-587S)

Riezzo G, Chiloiro M, Russo F. "Functional foods: salient features and clinical applications." *Curr Drug Targets Immune Endocr Metabol Disord.* (2005 Sep) 5(3):331-7.

Wolfe KL, Liu RH. "Apple peels as a value-added food ingredient." *J Agric Food Chem.* (2003 Mar 12) 51(6):1676-83.

Wolfe K, Wu X, Liu RH. "Antioxidant activity of apple peels." *J Agric Food Chem.* (2003 Jan 29) 51(3):609-14.

Yang CS, Lambert JD, Hou Z, Ju J, Lu G, Hao X. "Molecular targets for the cancer preventive activity of tea polyphenols." *Mol Carcinog.* (2006 Jun) 45(6):431-5.

CHAPTER 6 Myths and Facts about Food and Dieting

Berkey CS, Rockett HR, Willett WC, Colditz GA, "Milk, dairy fat, dietary calcium, and weight gain: a longitudinal study of adolescents." *Arch Pediatr Adolesc Med.* (2005 Jun) 159(6):543-50.

Brown MJ, Ferruzzi MG, Nguyen ML, Cooper DA, Eldridge AL, Schwartz SJ, White WS. "Carotenoid bioavailability is higher from salads ingested with full-fat than with fat-reduced salad dressings as measured with electrochemical detection." *Am J Clin Nutr.* (2004 Aug) 80(2):396-403.

Dewanto V, Wu X, Adom KK, Liu RH. "Thermal processing enhances the nutritional value of tomatoes by increasing total antioxidant activity." *J Agric Food Chem.* (2002 May 8) 50(10):3010-4

Fielding JM, Rowley KG, Cooper P, O' Dea K. "Increases in plasma lycopene concentration after consumption of tomatoes cooked with olive oil." *Asia Pac J Clin Nutr.* (2005) 14(2):131-6.

Harrison EH. "Mechanisms of digestion and absorption of dietary vitamin A." *Annu Rev Nutr.* (2005) 25:87-103.

Mulokozi G, Hedren E, Svanberg U. "In vitro accessibility and intake of beta-carotene from cooked green leafy vegetables and their estimated contribution to vitamin A requirements." *Plant Foods Hum Nutr.* (2004 Winter) 59(1):1-9.

Ribaya-Mercado JD. "Influence of dietary fat on beta-carotene absorption and bioconversion into vitamin A." *Nutr Rev.* (2002 Apr) 60(4):104-10.

Simopoulos AP. "The Mediterranean Diets: What Is So Special about the Diet of Greece? The Scientific Evidence." *J. Nutr.* (2001 Nov) 131:3065S-3073S.

Tang G, Ferreira AL, Grusak MA, Qin J, Dolnikowski GG, Russell RM, Krinsky NI. "Bioavailability of synthetic and biosynthetic deuterated lycopene in humans." *J Nutr Biochem.* (2005 Apr) 16(4):229-35.

Unlu NZ, Bohn T, Clinton SK, Schwartz SJ. "Carotenoid absorption from salad and salsa by humans is enhanced by the addition of avocado or avocado oil." *J Nutr.* (2005 Mar) 135(3):431-6.

CHAPTER 7 Why Wine Is Good For Your Diet

Alcocer F, Whitley D, Salazar-Gonzalez JF, Jordan WD, Sellers MT, Eckhoff DE, Suzuki K, Macrae C, Bland KI. "Quercetin inhibits human vascular smooth muscle cell proliferation and migration." *Surgery* (2002 Feb) 131(2):198-204.

Dashwood MR, Tsui JC. "Endothelins and the 'French paradox': are detrimental effects of red wine also associated with an action on endothelin synthesis?" *Angiology* (2002 Nov-Dec) 53(6):749-51.

de Lange DW. "From red wine to polyphenols and back: A journey through the history of the French Paradox." *Thromb Res.* (2006 Jul 11); [Epub ahead of print]

de Lorgeril M, Salen P, Paillard F, Laporte F, Boucher F, de Leiris J. "Mediterranean diet and the French paradox: two distinct biogeographic concepts for one consolidated scientific theory on the role of nutrition in coronary heart disease." *Cardiovasc Res.* (2002 Jun) 54(3):503-15.

Dixon JB, Dixon ME, O'Brien PE. "Reduced plasma homocysteine in obese red wine consumers: a potential contributor to reduced cardiovascular risk status." *Eur J Clin Nutr.* (2002 Jul) 56(7):608-14.

Dufour MC. "Risks and benefits of alcohol use over the life span." *Alcohol Health and Research World* (1996) 20:145-51.

Ferrieres J. "The French paradox: lessons for other countries." *Heart* (2004 Jan) 90(1):107-11.

Finkel H. "Wine's antioxidant assets." *The Wine News Magazine.* http://www.thewinenews.com/aprmay00/comment.html (accessed 2006 Sept).

"A glass of red wine a day keeps the doctor away." Nutrition Advisor, Yale-New Haven Hospital. http://www.ynhh.org/online/nutrition/advisor/red_wine.html (accessed 2006 Sept).

Gronbaek M. "Epidemiologic evidence for the cardioprotective effects associated with consumption of alcoholic beverages." *Pathophysiology* (2004 Apr) 10(2):83-92.

Howard A, Chopra M, Thurnham D, Strain J, Fuhrman B, Aviram M. "Red wine consumption and inhibition of LDL oxidation: what are the important components?" *Med Hypotheses* (2002 Jul) 59(1):101-4.

Iriti M, Faoro F. "Grape phytochemicals: A bouquet of old and new nutraceuticals for human health." *Med Hypotheses* (2006) 67(4):833-8. Epub (2006 Jun 8).

McCue K. "Wine Antioxidants." American Chemical Society. http://www.chemistry.org/portal/a/c/s/1/feature_pro.html?id=38d069c4dada11d5e4204fd8fe800100 (accessed 2006 Sept)

Poussier B, Cordova AC, Becquemin JP, Sumpio BE. "Resveratrol inhibits vascular smooth muscle cell proliferation and induces apoptosis." *J Vasc Surg.* (2005 Dec) 42(6):1190-7.

"Red Wine in Moderation Can Have a Positive Effect on Health." NCERx. http://www.red-wine-and-health.com/ (accessed 2006 Sept).

Renaud SC, Gueguen R, Schenker J, d'Houtaud A. "Alcohol and mortality in middle-aged men from eastern France." *Epidemiology* (1998) 9:184-8.

Rimm EB, Klatsky A, Grobbee D, Stampfer MJ. "Review of moderate alcohol consumption and reduced risk of coronary heart disease: is the effect due to beer, wine, or spirits." *BMJ* (1996) 312:731-6.

Rimm EB, Williams P, Fosher K, Criqui M, Stampfer MJ. "Moderate alcohol intake and lower risk of coronary heart disease: meta-analysis of effects on lipids and haemostatic factors." *BMJ* (1999) 319:1523-8.

Zern TL, Fernandez ML. "Cardioprotective effects of dietary polyphenols." *J Nutr.* (2005 Oct) 135(10):2291-4.

Index

About the Authors

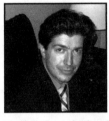

Apostolos Pappas, Ph.D., earned his Master of Science in Food Science and Nutrition and his doctorate in biochemistry. A research biochemist with Johnson & Johnson and a professional member of the Institute of Food Technology, he has received numerous awards and distinctions, including a Fulbright scholarship. Dr. Pappas's research and interests focus on lipid metabolism. A native of Greece, Dr. Pappas now lives in New York and New Jersey, where he enjoys his passions for cinema, music, and, of course, pairing his favorite wines to gourmet French meals.

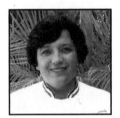

Marie-Annick Courtier is a native of Paris, France, where she grew up around gourmet foods and wines. Chef Marie holds a Culinary Arts Degree, has worked with many world-renowned chefs, and runs her own personal chef service. A Certified Fitness Nutritionist and Professional Food Manager, she also teaches cooking and created the new Certified Personal Fitness Chef Program marketed by Dr. John Spencer Ellis, president of the National Exercise & Sports Trainer Association (NESTA). Chef Marie lives in Orange County, California.

Visit us online at www.SaintTropezDiet.com.